Making Near-Death Experiences

A Handbook for Clinicians

EDITED BY

MAHENDRA PERERA, KARUPPIAH JAGADHEESAN AND ANTHONY PEAKE

FOREWORD BY JANICE HOLDEN

Jessica Kingsley *Publishers*
London and Philadelphia

The interview schedule and tape rating from Ring, 1980 on pp.138–149 are reproduced with permission of Dr Kenneth Ring. These questionnaires appeared in Ring, K. (1980) *Life at Death: A Scientific Investigation of the Near-Death Experience*. New York: Coward, McCann & Geoghegan.

The NDE scale on pp.150–152 is reproduced with permission of the International Association for Near-Death Studies. Reproduced with permission from Professor Bruce Greyson.

The NDE Questionnaire on p.153–154 is reproduced with permission from the principal author, Dr Mahendra Perera, and the Editor-in-chief, Janice Holden, *Journal of Near-Death Studies*. The questionnaire appeared in Perera, M., Padmasekara, G. and Belanti, J. (2005) 'Prevalence of near-death experiences in Australia.' *Journal of Near-Death Studies 24*, 109–116.

Chapter 5 is adapted from Miner *et al.* and reproduced with permission.

First published in 2012
by Jessica Kingsley Publishers
116 Pentonville Road
London N1 9JB, UK
and
400 Market Street, Suite 400
Philadelphia, PA 19106, USA

www.jkp.com

Copyright © Jessica Kingsley Publishers 2012
Foreword copyright © Janice Holden 2012

Library of Congress Cataloging in Publication Data
Making sense of near-death experiences : a handbook for clinicians / edited by
Mahendra Perera, Karuppiah Jagadheesan and Anthony Peake.
 p. cm.
 Includes bibliographical references and index.
 ISBN 978-1-84905-149-1 (alk. paper)
 1. Near-death experiences. 2. Near-death experiences--Psychological
aspects. I. Perera, Mahendra, 1951- II. Jagadheesan, Karuppiah, 1972- III.
Peake, Anthony.
 BF1045.N4M35 2012
 133.901'3--dc23
                            2011021216

British Library Cataloguing in Publication Data
A CIP catalogue record for this book is available from the British Library

ISBN 978 1 84905 149 1
eISBN 978 0 85700 342 3

Printed and bound in Great Britain

To those known and unknown who have gone before us and to all of us who will inevitably follow, for we are all one.

Contents

Foreword by Janice Holden   7

ACKNOWLEDGEMENTS   9

Introduction   11

Chapter 1   Near-Death Experiences: An Overview and
             Early Studies   17
             P.M.H. Atwater, Retired investigative researcher
             and author

Chapter 2   A Critical Review of Epidemiological
             Studies of Near-Death Experiences, 2001–2010   24
             Mahendra Perera, Albert Road Clinic, Melbourne
             and Rohan Jayasuriya, University of New South Wales

Chapter 3   Phenomenology of Near-Death Experiences   36
             Karuppiah Jagadheesan, North West Area Mental
             Health Service, Victoria and John Belanti, North
             West Area Mental Health Service, Victoria

Chapter 4   Dealing with Diversity: Cross-Cultural
             Aspects of Near-Death Experiences   51
             Ornella Corazza, University of Hertfordshire and
             K.A.L.A. Kuruppuarachchi, University of Kelaniya

Chapter 5   Near-Death Experiences of Children   63
             Cherie Sutherland, researcher, educator and sociologist

Chapter 6   Pathophysiological Aspects of Near-Death
             Experiences   79
             Pim van Lommel, Cardiologist, Hospital Rijnstate,
             Arnhem, The Netherlands

Chapter 7   Psychological Aspects of Near-Death
Experiences   94

Satwant K. Pasricha, Former Professor and
Chair, National Institute of Mental Health and
Neorosciences, Department of Clinical Psychology,
Bangalore

Chapter 8   Light and Near-Death Experiences   103
Anthony Peake, Giordano Bruno University

Chapter 9   Religious Significance of Near-Death
Experiences   117
Paul Badham, Emeritus Professor of Theology and
Religious Studies, University of Wales

Chapter 10   Assessment and Management of Near-
Death Experiences   122
Peter Fenwick, Institute of Psychiatry, London

Chapter 11   Prospecting in the Light: The Future of
Near-Death Experiences Research   128
David J. Wilde, University of Manchester, and
Craig D. Murray, Lancaster University

Conclusion   135

APPENDIX 1: INTERVIEW SCHEDULE   138

APPENDIX 2: TAPE RATING FORM   144

APPENDIX 3: NEAR-DEATH EXPERIENCE SCALE   150

APPENDIX 4: NDE QUESTIONNAIRE   153

THE CONTRIBUTORS   155

REFERENCES   160

SUBJECT INDEX   172

AUTHOR INDEX   175

Foreword

In a recent study of 109 upper level undergraduate students at a large Southwestern US university (Holden, Oden, Kozlowski and Hayslip 2011), participants answered 20 questions about near-death experiences (NDEs). The questions addressed facts that 35 years of research on NDEs have established. Possible response to each question ranged from 1 (strongly disagree) to 4 (uncertain) to 7 (strongly agree). Participants' average score was 4.74 – somewhat better than an average of 4 if students had acknowledged uncertainty or were randomly guessing, but far below a perfect score of 7. Despite the fact that, to date, more than 65 NDE research studies have been published involving over 3500 near-death experiencers in the US, Europe, Asia, and Australia and focusing on the experience itself and/or its aftereffects (Holden, Greyson and James 2009), and despite increasing media coverage of NDEs and online availability of NDE narratives, widespread absence of information and misinformation about NDEs persist.

The nature of this need for accurate information begins with a most fundamental point: the difference between a near-death *episode* and a near-death *experience*. The confusion occurs when any close brush with death – a near-death episode – is referred to as a near-death experience – which actually is a subjective experience reported by only about a quarter of all people who survive a close brush with death (Zingrone and Alvarado 2009). Near-death experiencers typically say that at the point that their bodies were near or actually in the first moments of death, their consciousness, now separated from their physical bodies, continued to experience and perceive the material world and/or a transmaterial domain of environments and entities. Many journalists unfortunately perpetuate the confusion by referring to any near-death episode as a near-death experience.

In the aftermath of NDEs, experiencers may turn to health care providers for understanding, information and assistance. However, a recent review of research indicated that 'medical and spiritual health care providers are only somewhat familiar with NDEs and that what they do know seems only partially accurate' – despite positive attitudes toward NDEs and a desire to learn more about them (Foster, James and Holden 2009, p. 256).

Undergraduates, journalists and health care providers all point to the need for resources that familiarize and inform about NDEs. *Making Sense of Near-Death Experiences* offers readers just such a resource. Chapter authors reflect an international span, representing the US, Europe, and Asia. With works by veteran researchers in the field such as mental health therapist Cherie Sutherland, cardiologist Pim van Lommel, and neuropsychiatrist Peter Fenwick, along with NDE scholars from the UK and India, readers hear many voices and are exposed to many perspectives on NDEs. Readers encounter both already-known information from, and also future-projected directions in, NDE investigation through chapters that range from general overviews to specific technical treatises. For readers whose interest is piqued to pursue further inquiry through primary and other quality secondary sources, *Making Sense of Near-Death Experiences* points such readers to many of those sources.

Even as a veteran near-death researcher, I found *Making Sense of Near-Death Experiences* an interesting and provocative read. I believe readers will come away from this book with not only an understanding of diverse viewpoints about NDEs but also an awareness of the complexity of the field of near-death studies and an appreciation for the value of continued research in the field. Thus the title *Making Sense of Near-Death Experiences* indicates appropriately not only a review of what is already known of NDEs so far but also an endeavor for humanity to continue pursuing into the future.

Janice Holden, Ed.D., LPC-S, LMFT, NCC
Professor, Counseling Program
Chair, Department of Counseling and Higher Education
University of North Texas, USA

Acknowledgements

We are sincerely grateful to all of those who made this venture a success by contributing in many different ways, including the authors who gave tirelessly of their time and the publication staff at Jessica Kingsley Publishers. A special word of thanks to Caroline Walton of JKP who responded to our many questions in a timely manner.

Dr Bruce Greyson has helped us in many ways in the pursuit of this work and provided timely advice, necessary literature from his collection and permission to reproduce the NDE Scale. Dr Janice Holden, the Editor of the *Journal of Near-Death Studies* helped us by swift and helpful responses to our email queries and allowing us to reproduce the NDE Questionnaire.

Dr Kenneth Ring was gracious in his response to our request and extended his permission to reproduce both the interview schedule and the tape rating form of Weighted Core Experience Index Scale.

Chapter 5, 'Near-Death Experiences of Children' is abridged from the chapter 'Trailing Clouds of Glory: The Near-Death Experiences of Western Children and Teens', in *The Handbook of Near-Death Experiences: Thirty Years of Investigation* (edited by Janice Miner Holden, Bruce Greyson and Debbie James). We thank the editors and the publisher for permission to use material from the original chapter.

The empirical research quoted in Chapter 11 was supported by the Bial Foundation, a Parapsychological Association Research Endowment, and also, in part, by a Faculty Scholarship Fund granted by the Faculty of Medical and Human Sciences at the University of Manchester. David Wilde and Craig Murray would like to express their gratitude in this regard.

We sincerely appreciate those who shared their personal stories about near-death experiences that have been cited in this book. Without this information, the purpose of this book would not have been achieved.

We graciously acknowledge that much time was taken away from family commitments while we were busy with collating and editing the contributions. Finally this acknowledgement will not be complete unless

I (Mahendra Perera) personally thank one individual who has tirelessly and without returns worked behind the scenes, perhaps not even knowing he was helping at times. He is my dear uncle in Sri Lanka, P.A.D. Perera, who has been a tower of strength and helped me to bring together the material in a meaningful and timely manner.

Introduction

It is not all of life to live nor all of death to die. (Edgar Cayce, 1877–1945)

This book was born of a desire to promote a broader understanding of near-death experiences (NDEs) among the range of professionals who are likely to encounter clients or patients who have had such an experience. In this book, we consider NDEs as unusual experiences that are experienced by some individuals who have been faced with situations that are potentially fatal, or have been in states of unconsciousness, which in some situations are artificially induced (e.g. aneasthesia). On the other hand a near-death episode is one in which the individual faces a similar situation but does not recall or relate any experience. They would say, "there is nothing".

A universal definition of NDE has yet to be established, but in this book we attempt to give a detailed definition as provided by research workers in Chapter 2, dealing with epidemiology.

Briefly, it is a relatively common phenomenon: the consensus suggests that there are about 4 to 8 per cent in a general population and about one in five who have faced potentially fatal situations who have had an NDE (of course, this means that there will be many who have not had the experience).

People who have had this experience in general report a sense of transcendence. They claim it is a mystical experience, with different aspects being reported by different individuals. A feeling of unity with a cosmic consciousness is reported by some and some individuals have physical effects such as wrist watches not keeping to time when they now wear these: some even report foreknowledge of future events. There are, however, others who have been distressed by certain things that they have seen or felt during their NDEs and others who, due to giving up on material benefits or seeing the world through different eyes, get disheartened by existential realities and suffer with low mood, relationship problems and the like.

Dr Raymond Moody Jr is probably one of the most cited authors in the field and he spurred a deeper interest in the phenomenon with the publication of his book *Life After Life* in 1975. He also coined the term 'near-death experience'. More details of the events that led to the seminal work of Dr Moody are provided in Chapter 1.

Dr Moody studied philosophy at the University of Virginia, US, where he obtained a BA (1966), an MA (1967) and a PhD (1969) in the subject. He also obtained a PhD in psychology from the University of West Georgia, then known as West Georgia College, where he later became a professor in that topic. He then studied medicine and specialized in psychiatry. In 1976, he was awarded an MD from the Medical College of Georgia.

Two other key figures in the field are Professor Bruce Greyson and Dr Kenneth Ring. Professor Greyson MD is a Founder and long-time Research Director of the International Association for Near-Death Studies (IANDS) and was for more than two decades Editor-in-Chief of the *Journal of Near-Death Studies*. Dr Ring, PhD is Professor Emeritus of psychology at the University of Connecticut, and a researcher within the field of near-death studies. He is co-founder and past president of the IANDS and is the founding editor of the *Journal of Near-Death Studies*. Dr Elisabeth Kübler-Ross, a psychiatrist better known for her work on death and dying, has also studied NDE.

My journey (Mahendra Perera) into this field began in 1976 as a young house officer who spotted Moody's book *Life After Life* in a bookstore in Colombo, Sri Lanka. Due to financial constraints, I was unable to purchase it and so I wrote to the author who kindly mailed me a copy and corresponded with me. Many years later this book remains a treasured item on my bookshelf. Many decades later when I corresponded with Dr Moody he said he remembered the deed. The esoteric aspects of life always appealed to me but I try as far as possible to retain a questioning mind when delving into the unfolding mysteries and the existential dilemmas of life. There were unexpected or coincidental meetings with my colleagues; perhaps the most influential in regard to the book was that the co-editors shared the burden of the endeavour.

The field of near-death studies is replete with written material. There are many personal anecdotes as well as articles in the popular press and scientific journals. There are numerous books dealing with the subject, which include poignant and instructive narratives. In addition scholarly text have been published. There are those who question the veracity of the reports and attempt to portray NDE in narrowly scientific and reductionist terms. Others may be accused of being too willing to accept without question every whit and jot that has been told as 'gospel'. However one may view the phenomenon, it is the reality of the experience to the experiencer and the effect it has on their lives that are our primary concerns. Clinicians, healing professionals, are held in regard and esteem by patients. NDEs occur usually in life-threatening situations and the first contact could well be a nurse, doctor or an allied health professional. Human beings like to tell their story, especially of an unusual experience and hope that the health care giver will be able to help the individual and to make sense of what he/she thinks has happened. Unfortunately the topic of NDEs is not well understood nor taught in the curricula (to the best of our knowledge) in routine teaching of health care givers. The account is therefore discounted, labelled as hallucinations or worse, or perhaps benignly and politely ignored. Our aim in writing this text is to help introduce the topic primarily to clinicians but it is not necessarily limited to an academic audience. We hope that this book will help 'NDErs' (people who have had an NDE) and significant others in the life of the NDEr, and others who are interested or have a healthy degree of scepticism. Common features of NDEs are well known and documented and are reiterated in the material to follow. There is debate in relation to the underlying physiological and psychological bases to the phenomena and they are also discussed.

As editors, we began this endeavour with a view to striking a balance between strictly scientific work and merely presenting a point of view and we hope that we have achieved this – we will let the reader be the judge. We hope the book will help not only clinicians who have begun training but also more senior personnel who would like to understand what might seem to be an unusual experience among their clients. In addition it is our intention that this book will be of use to anyone who has an interest in or has had an NDE.

Although each chapter has a different focus, given the nature of the topic there is some degree of overlap in the material presented, demonstrating internal consistency of views expressed by different authors.

The book begins with a chapter from P.M.H. Atwater, who has had NDEs and is a published author on NDE. She gives us a broad overview of NDE as an NDEr and shares her own personal knowledge with the reader. The chapter also highlights another less well known aspect of NDE – that of the experience of groups and shared NDEs. The shared and group NDEs open exciting vistas regarding the underlying explanations for NDE and take us further afield in relation to what an NDE may be or indeed whether the shared and group experiences need to be looked upon as related but not central to NDE. However, these issues are beyond the ambit of the present work. Atwater concludes the chapter by noting the transformational changes, mainly of a positive nature, that follow NDEs.

How many have NDEs and how is this assessed? These are the aspects discussed in Chapter 2. In writing this chapter, Mahendra Perera was ably assisted by an epidemiologist, Rohan Jayasuriya. A survey of the literature reveals that it is not a rare event and has been reported from various parts of the globe. However, further development in terms of research techniques and application is shown to be in order.

Karuppiah Jagadheesan and John Belanti expand further on the nature of NDEs as well as explore other situations where NDE-like states may occur and finally give the readers some questionnaires that have been used in NDE research (Chapter 3).

Ornella Corraza and K.A.L.A. Kuruppuarachchi (Chapter 4) take us on a tour of NDEs as reported from different parts of the globe. Aptly called 'Dealing with diversity: cross-cultural aspects of NDEs' the chapter gives various accounts and concludes by comparing the prototypical 'Western' model with that of the 'non-Western' type and outlining clinical relevance.

Cherie Sutherland, a counsellor who has written several books primarily dealing with the NDEs of children, has made the contribution regarding the experiences of children of all ages and teenagers (Chapter 5). By relating the stories of NDErs, she has succeeded in giving the reader an inside view into the children's experiences. She also refers to the pioneering work done by Dr Melvin Morse, a peadiatrician who has studied NDEs in children since 1980. The chapter not only educates the reader about how children could be helped but also shows how a grieving adult may find solace from the children's narratives.

Pim van Lommel, a Dutch cardiologist and researcher, has helped us to explore the underlying biological bases (Chapter 6). He has examined various physical and physiological bases that could possibly explain what happens when one has an NDE. He then looks beyond a reductionist scientific paradigm in terms of the phenomenon.

Psychological aspects of NDE (Chapter 7) is the next offering and is provided by Satwant Pasricha from India. NDEs from the subcontinent have been utilized to illustrate her teaching. She has provided psychological tenets but above all gives advice on how to help the NDEr.

Anthony Peake takes a different approach to an explanatory model of NDEs (Chapter 8). He draws on studies from Austria in which light has been a central feature in treating disturbed children and then speculates once more on neuro-chemical bases, which will assist in transmitting knowledge from another dimensions, the knowledge that is being channelled via unknown or occult source. He ends the chapter with the rhetorical question: what is real?

Paul Badham has given us an overview of NDEs from the perspective of contemporary and ancient religious practices (Chapter 9). Looking at religious creeds, he considers motifs that could be interpreted as 'evidence' of near-death phenomena, illustrating the common thread of the different religious teachings. Finally he ponders on the question of continuity of life.

Peter Fenwick, in Chapter 10, adopts a medical model in the process of assessment of NDEs. He argues for the need for investigations when appropriate. He also brings into focus a related matter, that is, end-of-life experiences. These are akin to NDEs and are related by patients mainly in palliative care settings. This is a topic of relevance to clinicians, and knowledge and understanding of it helps grieving relatives and friends in not too dissimilar circumstances to those discussed by Cherie Sutherland.

Craig Murray and David Wilde write in the final chapter (Chapter 11) about the future of NDE research. They examine research work to date and open up areas for future research work on NDEs. They too critically evaluate studies, as has been done in the chapter on epidemiology (Chapter 2), thereby giving guidance for future work. Furthermore, they critically evaluate the existing models of phenomenology (or theoretical models). Some of these models have been covered in the phenomenology chapter (Chapter 3).

Many of the authors have noted the ephemeral nature of the experience, and the overall sense of well-being. Remarkable similarities have been seen across different cultural, ethnic and religious groups. There is almost a mystical nature in the field of NDE studies. There are many and varied views on the genesis of NDE. The authors who contributed have presented their points of view and our aim in presenting this work is to keep an open mind. Each step in the journey will help us in gaining a better understanding leading to greater help for the person who has had an NDE and struggles to make sense of what they perceive has taken place.

It is our sincere hope that readers will gain a broader understanding of the concept. There are many leads for those interested to follow. There is unlimited scope for pursuing various lines of enquiry.

CHAPTER 1

Near-Death Experiences

An Overview and Early Studies

P.M.H. ATWATER

There is more to life than we think there is, and more to death
than finality. (P.M.H. Atwater)

Objective studies of reports from those who died or nearly died,
experienced what they believed to have been life on the other side of
death, then revived, were published as early as 1825 (a few more have
surfaced with even earlier dates). In 1975 the publication of *Life After
Life*, by Raymond A. Moody, Jr, MD, PhD popularized the concept and
introduced the phrase 'near-death experience' (NDE) (Moody 1975).
Elisabeth Kübler-Ross, MD, backed up his work with her own (Kübler-
Ross 1991).

What initially inspired Moody to explore this 'strange phenomenon'
was a talk he heard given by George Ritchie, in Charlottesville, Virginia.
Ritchie had contracted double pneumonia as a 20-year-old US Army
private and was pronounced dead, his corpse taken to the base morgue.
Nine minutes later, after what seemed to him to be lengthy visits in other
worlds, Ritchie chose to return – but couldn't find his body in a room
filled with corpses covered by sheets. A hand hung below one of the
sheets wearing Ritchie's class ring. An orderly passing by the room saw

that hand suddenly wiggle and rushed to find a physician. A shot of adrenaline restarted vital signs. Later on he became a psychiatrist (Ritchie and Sherill 1978).

Concerned by all the media publicity generated by his book, Moody invited a number of researchers from across the country to meet with him in Charlottesville during the weekend of 17 November 1977. To make their goal official, they agreed to incorporate under the banner, Association for the Scientific Study of Near-Death Phenomena, which later on became the International Association for Near-Death Studies (IANDS). Near-death studies as a legitimate field of enquiry was born that day, fuelled for several decades to come first by Kenneth Ring, PhD, who scientifically verified Moody's work in his seminal book *Life at Death* (1980), and then by Bruce Greyson, MD and Charles Flynn, PhD, with *The Near-Death Experience: Problems, Prospects, Perspectives* (1984). Although many researchers have expanded the field with their work, Greyson remains to this day the one who has published the most papers. (Greyson and Flynn 1984; Kelly, Greyson and Kelly 2007) and Ring (Ring 1980, 1982, 1984; Ring and Valarino 2006)

I entered the picture in 1981 after Ring purchased a self-published piece called *I Died Three Times in 1977* (Atwater 1980) at a Connecticut bookstore. He discovered that I had been researching near-death states independently since 1978, after learning about them from Kübler-Ross. It was because of what a 'voice' told me during my third NDE that I became a researcher.

What began in Charlottesville has now encircled the globe, inspiring researchers, clinicians, scholars, educators, clerics, people from every walk of life in every discipline – not to mention the millions upon millions of experiencers – newborns, babies, toddlers, children and teens of every age, adults and seniors of every race, job history, educational level, culture, philosophical bent, and financial advantage or disadvantage. It is the author's contention that NDE having captured the world's attention, studies and research on the near-death phenomenon have directly impinged on what we think and know about the capacity of the human mind and spirit, our religious and social structures, and the prospect of life after death, for example moving away from religious dogmas, and becoming less materialistic and more spiritual (van Lommel 2010; Ring and Valarino 2006).

This definition of near-death was developed by IANDS and was used by them for many years:

> an intense awareness, sense, or experience of otherworldliness, whether pleasant or unpleasant, that happens to people who are at the edge of death. It is of such magnitude that the vast majority are deeply affected, many to the point of making significant changes in their lives afterward because of what they went through.*

Although it is true that the closer people are to physical death the more apt they are to have one, 'near-death-like' experiences can occur without the threat of imminent death. Drugs, oxygen deprivation, temporal lobe seizures, psychological disorders, and other possible mediators, have all been considered as probable etiologic factors. However, none of these conditions account for the full range of experiences (van Lommel 2010).

A signature feature of the phenomenon is that no matter how long an experiencer is without vital signs – no pulse, no breath, no indicators of brainwave activity – not only will little or no brain damage be found, but, on average, individuals once revived or resuscitated will begin to display an unexplainable enhancement of intellect (van Lommel 2010).

To quote the Dutch cardiologist, Pim van Lommel, MD: 'How could clear, continuous consciousness – outside one's body – be experienced at the moment that the brain no longer functions during a period of clinical death, with a flat EEG?' (van Lommel 2005). This is the enigma faced by all medical practitioners: the wakeful activity of brain and perceptual faculties when the organ shuts down in a flatline. The range of that activity and the pattern of after-effects which follow suggest changes in the brain/mind assembly, nervous system, digestive system, and skin sensitivity that defies what can presently be explained or understood.

As concerns the original model of the experience itself, Moody (1975) identified 15 elements overall: ineffability (beyond the limits of any language to describe), hearing yourself pronounced dead, feelings of peace and quiet, hearing unusual noises, seeing a dark tunnel, finding yourself outside your body, meeting 'spiritual beings', a very bright light experienced as a 'being of light', a panoramic life review, sensing a border or limit to where you can go, coming back into your body, frustrating attempts to tell others about what happened to you, subtle 'broadening and deepening' of your life afterward, elimination of the fear of death,

---

* See www.iands.org/about-ndes/key-nde-facts.html. Accessed 17 April 2011.

and corroboration of events witnessed while out of your body. After hundreds more interviews, Moody added four more elements to what experiencers claimed to have encountered: a realm where all knowledge exists, cities of light, a realm of bewildered spirits, and supernatural rescues (Moody 1975).

This 'classical model' is now subject to revision. People in many countries, for instance, never mention tunnels or life reviews or cities of light. In the first Gallup Poll Survey done in the US 15 per cent said yes to the question 'Have you, yourself, ever been on the verge of death or had a "close call" which involved any unusual experience at that time?' (Gallup and Proctor 1982, p.200). Of those who responded yes (i.e.15%) there were 3 per cent who described a 'perception of a tunnel' making it 20 per cent reporting anything like a tunnel (p.201). In my own work, I never found that 'elements' defined how simple, complex, or deep an experience was. Rather, I discovered four scenario patterns that consistently addressed the spread of what individuals experienced. These are:

- *Initial* – like an awakening (always brief, maybe one to three elements, such as the loving nothingness, the living dark, a friendly voice, a brief out-of-body experience, a manifestation of some type)

- *Unpleasant or Hellish* – like an inner cleansing, self-confrontational experience (encounter with a threatening void, stark limbo, hellish purgatory, scenes of a startling indifference, haunting from one's own past)

- *Pleasant or Heavenly* – like self-validation, reassurance (loving family reunions, reassuring religious figures or light beings, validation that life counts, affirmative and inspiring dialogue, being guided by angels, religious figures, pets)

- *Transcendent* – alternate realities, expansive revelations (exposure to other-worldly dimensions, scenes beyond the individual's frame of reference, revelations of greater truths – seldom personal in content, more concerned with the human/spiritual collective).

It is of interest to note that in the research I did most cases with women arose from crises involving birth, miscarriage, rape, or hysterectomies.

But with men, most of them were heart-related or resulted from acts of violence or accidents. With children, it was birth trauma or accidents, often involving a drowning or suffocation; some were from surgery and situations of abuse (Atwater 2007). This is basically what other researchers have encountered as well.

After-effects are far more involved and in-depth than at first thought. The pattern of psychological changes is well known. But the physiological pattern is just now becoming more recognized and accepted. Here are some of the changes with percentages from my work, to offer perspective: between 80 and 90 per cent claimed to look and act younger, and were more playful afterward. They evidenced brighter skin, eyes that sparkled, and said there were substantial changes in their energy levels (even energy surges). They spoke of increased sensitivity to light and especially sunlight, increased sensitivity to sound and noise levels, a regard for things as new even when they weren't, decreased boredom levels, stress being easier to handle, healing more quickly, changes in intelligence levels, and becoming 'creative intuitives' (Atwater and Morgan 2000).

Seventy-three per cent experienced electrical sensitivity, where their personal biofield (subtle energy field that permeates the living body) affected the electromagnetic fields around them – such as with computers, television sets, tape recorders, security systems, microphones, light bulbs, watches, and so forth. Indications that their energy seems to interfere with or enhance the performance of technological equipment and batteries are typical.

Well over half reported metabolic changes that affected their digestion and ability to assimilate substances, such as pharmaceuticals (Atwater and Morgan 2000). Drug tolerance decreased, as it took less of something to obtain full effect. Allergies heightened, especially to chemical additives, strong smells, and pollutants. Blood pressure lowered. Body clocks tended to reverse, with incidents of waking up around 3:00 am feeling unusually creative or uplifted fairly frequent. Dreams became more vivid. Claims of conjoined senses (synaesthesia) were common, along with heightened sensations and cognitive abilities that seem to switch in function.

Certainly, clinical tests are needed to measure the full import of after-effects. Initial research, however, is highly suggestive that a pattern of physiological and psychological changes is indeed valid and real. There are medical schools that offer classes on the near-death phenomenon (e.g. Sheeler 2005). I am advised of one incident where medical foreknowledge of the NDE made a difference. In 2008, a child experiencer, now adult, was rushed to John Hopkins Hospital with complications from lupus. She told the attending physician that she had had an NDE when seven years old. The physician wanted to know more. After hearing her story, he changed her medication and dosage to the mildest possible. She recovered so quickly she was sent home the next day and has yet to have a recurrence. This physician knew about near-death after-effects and that the majority lose their tolerance of pharmaceuticals afterward. His alertness proved crucial.

Children and adults experience the same pattern of episode scenarios and after-effects, but they respond differently. The average adult takes between seven and ten years to integrate their experience, but most child experiencers take at least 20 to 30 years. Why so long? Children compensate, they do not integrate. They adjust their lives in accord with life events, seldom 'connecting the dots' of cause and effect. Many times, a child will repress or 'tuck away' their experience should they be made fun of in the telling of their story. After-effects can be denied, explained away, or called something else, but not hidden. The areas where children are challenged the most are in school and in social events. In those homes where parents are more open or knowledgeable, kids not only do well but their differences often lead to decided advantages in career choices, the creative arts, and intuitive awareness.

Any knee-jerk reaction to research findings, or to the idea that we alone decide our heavens and hells based on personal beliefs and attitudes, falls apart when we examine shared and group experiences.

Shared near-death states*

There are cases in which several experiencers seem to share in each other's episode, that is to say they have the same or similar elements, scenario type, or basic storyline. These are usually encountered when two or three

---

*   See also You Tube video of an interview with Dr Raymond Moody available at www. youtube.com/watch?v=DvNDrZv8HwE&feature=youtu.be. Accessed 17 April 2011.

people are involved in the same accident at the same time, or are in the same general section of the hospital at the same time. Sometimes these states are experienced singly (one individual is not aware of the other during the episode, but later learns that both apparently experienced the same scenario). Sometimes the people involved are aware of each other, and are able to confirm the extent of that awareness, after they compare their separate stories (Atwater 2007).

Group near-death states

These are rare, but they do occur (Atwater 2007). With this type, a whole group of people simultaneously seems to experience the same or similar episode. What makes these so spectacular and challenging is that all or most of the experiencers see each other actually leave their bodies as this occurs, then dialogue with each other and share messages and observations while still in the near-death state. Their separate reports afterward either exactly or nearly match. Such reports emerge most often from events of a harrowing nature that involve a number of people (e.g. a crew of fire fighters who suffocated *en masse*).

Shared and group experiences imply that no matter how sure we are that near-death states mean this or that, and are the result of whatever, no single idea, theory, or glib answer can explain them. Even clues from the powerful patterning those researchers like myself have identified fail to explain all aspects of the phenomenon.

Experiencers of NDEs report a wide array of phenomena, which are not easily explicable with the known science of today. Most have positive transformative changes which impact on their lives. They speak of wanting to make a difference in society, love and oneness and about God, Allah or another deity.

A Critical Review of Epidemiological Studies of Near-Death Experiences, 2001–2010

MAHENDRA PERERA AND ROHAN JAYASURIYA

Introduction

Epidemiology is the science for the study of distributions and determinants of disease, illness and disability in populations. These methods can be very usefully applied to most conditions and states that humans face. The near-death experience (NDE) is no exception. A central tenet used in epidemiology is understanding of the characteristics and interactions between the host (in this case humans), environment (external factors) and the vector (situations that transmit or exacerbate).

Epidemiological studies follow a certain sequence when new diseases or conditions are investigated. Often these conditions first come to the attention of astute clinicians, who observe unusual occurrences and communicate these as individual or a series of case studies. This is usually followed by a flurry of research to 'measure' the frequency of the phenomenon. This requires the identification of inclusion and exclusion criteria to count a 'case'. In the case of NDE, much of the interest began following Raymond Moody's work in which he described the phenomenon that people frequently experience when coming close to dying. Based on about 50 people who were interviewed, Moody demonstrated the occurrence of what he named as 'near-death experience' (Moody 1975). Ring (1980) identified five stages to be the 'core experience' and constructed a scale to help quantify the phenomenon. This scale was called the Weighted Core Experience Index (WCEI) Scale. Subsequently another scale was constructed by Greyson (1983), which was called the Near-Death Experience Scale (NDES). He notes, 'For research purposes, the criterion score of 7 or higher (1 SD (standard deviation) below the mean) seems a valid cut-off point for selecting a group of subjects with NDEs for further study' (p.375). These scales are reproduced as appendices at the end of the book.

Assessing NDE

The NDE itself was conceptualized as 'an altered state of consciousness occurring during an episode of unconsciousness resulting from severe trauma or other life-threatening condition, in which a series of well-defined characteristics are present' (Greyson 1983, p.369). Olson and Dulaney (1993) operationalized the definition of NDE as 'It is identified by self-report on a questionnaire using standard questions and by content analysis of anecdotal data using the NDES with a score of seven as an indication of a near-death experience' (p.369).

After a phenomenon has been described, epidemiological techniques are used to measure the frequency of its occurrence in populations and to find specific characteristics of the host and environment that are associated with it. These studies usually use observational epidemiological techniques such as cross-sectional studies (where data is gathered at one or multiple points) and cohort studies (where identified groups of respondents are followed up over time). A measure of disease frequency needs to take into account the size of the source population from which the affected individuals were derived. This can be expressed as a ratio, the numbers of cases to the size of the source population, or as a rate. A rate is strictly speaking a ratio where a measure of time is applied to both the numerator and denominator, for instance the number of NDE in one year divided by the mid-year source population. The measures of frequency of a condition used in epidemiology fall into two categories: prevalence or incidence. The former allows us to measure the 'prevalence' (all new and old cases) of a condition and the latter is used to measure 'incidence'(new occurrences). In medical and public health literature, prevalence is used in two ways:

- Point Prevalence: number of affected persons in the population at a specific point of time.

- Period Prevalence: number of affected persons in the population over a certain period of time, such as a calendar year.

Another measure, not often used, is 'cumulative incidence', in which we find out the total number of cases that ever had the disease or condition. This is illustrated when one asks in a survey of a given population 'Have you ever had NDE?' (Gordis 2008).

When the duration of disease, such as an episode of NDE, is limited to a very short period of time the numerator (cases of NDE) for calculation of incidence and point prevalence (prevalence at one point of time) are the same. In the case of NDE, even the period prevalence rate (over one year) is the same as incidence rate. Therefore we use the term 'incidence' to denote both in this chapter. Table 2.1 shows wide variation in the estimates of incidence.

Over the period 1980–1998, there were many studies of incidence of NDE, which had a wide variation in results. Greyson (1998) reviewed all published studies and came to the conclusions that there was:

- a need to have consensus on the definition of NDE

- a need to obtain better representativeness of study sample to the study population

- a need for recognition of publication bias

- a need for studies on the trends of NDE frequency.

The purpose of this chapter is to provide clinicians with a critical review of the methodological aspects of studies in NDE, and in particular studies that have ascertained the frequency of NDE in populations around the

Table 2.1: Published studies included in the review 2001–2010

Year	First author	Source of study subjects and country	Measure of NDE	No of cases/at-risk population	Estimated incidence (%)
2001	Knoblauch	National survey, Germany	Researcher developed	82/356	23.0
2001	Parnia	Cardiac arrest, Southampton Hospital, UK	NDES	4/63	6.3
2001	van Lommel	Cardiac arrest, ten hospitals in Netherlands	WCEI	62/344	18.0
2002	Schwaninger	Cardiac arrest, one hospital, US	WCEI and NDE	7/30	23.3
2003	Greyson	Cardiac cases, one hospital, US	NDES	11/116	9.5
2003	Greyson	Psychiatry clinic, outpatient clinic, one hospital, US	NDES	61/272	22.4
2006	Greyson	Induced cardiac arrest, one hospital, US	NDES	unknown	0
2006	Perera	National survey, Australia	Items from NDES	60/673	8.9
2007	Lai	Renal dialysis, seven centres, Taiwan	NDES and WCEI	45/710	6.3
2008	Kuruppuarachchi	Attempted suicide, one hospital, Sri Lanka	NDES	0/77	0
2008	Pasricha	India in households	Questions	21/36,100	0.06*
2010	Corazza	Ketamine users, students, University, UK	NDES	50/125	40.0
2010	Kelmenc-Ketis	Cardiac arrest, three hospitals, Slovenia	NDES	11/52	21.5
2010	Fracasso	Iranian Moslem University students	NDES and questions	19/30**	63

NDES = Near-Death Experience Scale (Greyson, 1983); WCEI = Weighted Core Experience Index (Ring 1980)

*Our calculation based on the figures presented yield 0.06%. The value quoted in the paper is 4 per 10,000 (Pasricha 2008, p.267)

**These were from people who reported a brush with death and claimed to remember some events.

world and studies that have sought the aetiology of NDE. This chapter will present methods of critical appraisal relevant to NDE studies and use a set of criteria to appraise recent (2001–2010) studies conducted to measure frequency and aetiology of NDE (Table 2.1). We reviewed the current literature over the last ten years so that the conclusions generated could be contemporary. Using the appraisal method, bias in studies will be identified and described. Finally this chapter will discuss gaps in the evidence and potential areas for future research.

Methods of critical appraisal for studies of frequency and aetiology

Types of epidemiological study designs

DESCRIPTIVE STUDIES

Descriptive studies describe the pattern of disease occurrence in relation to variables such as person, place and time. Case studies, correlational studies and cross-sectional studies belong to this group. Of relevance for NDE research are cross-sectional studies, especially those undertaken to ascertain the frequency of NDE. Cross-sectional design is used to assess exposure to a situation and NDE simultaneously, usually using survey techniques in populations. As both exposure and disease are assessed at a single point of time it is difficult to determine whether the exposure always preceded NDE. Perhaps more importantly the design also suffers from recall bias if it is based on reports in the past. The most useful information obtained from such studies is 'period prevalence', the number of cases in a given period of time, which can be used to find relationship to characteristics of the person, place and trends over time.

ANALYTICAL STUDIES

These are designed to answer questions of aetiology (determinants) of disease and can be divided into observational studies and experimental studies. In the latter, researchers assign the interventions to the groups. Two major types of epidemiological designs for observational studies are case control studies and cohort studies. Subjects (cases of NDE) are selected based on strict criteria and compared with non-cases (controls or those without NDE) to ascertain the frequency of an exposure. They are efficient in the study of characteristics of NDE as NDE is not a common condition. As both exposure (to risk such as cardiac arrest) and outcome (NDE) have taken place prior to the investigation, they are sometimes called retrospective studies, a term better left for a type of cohort studies. These studies are prone to recall bias in measurement of both exposure and outcome.

Cohort studies overcome some of the above shortcomings, as one starts with a population (cohort) without NDE, but who have differential exposure to risk. In addition the temporal sequence between the exposure and disease can be evaluated. Cohort studies are classified as either prospective or retrospective. Prospective cohort design has since 2001 become the standard for NDE studies, as it allows the researchers to collect data to reduce recall bias. In retrospective studies all relevant events (exposure and disease) have already occurred when the study is initiated. Retrospective cohort studies have the advantage of time and cost efficiency. Therefore these studies are useful for conditions with long latency, which is not the case for NDE. In some instances a cohort study is ambidirectional: data is collected both retrospectively and prospectively in the same cohort. An additional modification of the cohort design is a nested case control study in either a retrospective or prospective study (Gordis 2008).

Critical appraisal of epidemiological studies

The purpose of critical appraisal is to ascertain if the findings of a study are reliable, valid and generalizable to populations of interest. Internal validity of a study considers whether the findings are true and accurate, while generalizability considers external validity of the findings. Internal validity can be classified to consist of systematic error and random error (see Table 2.2). The key questions that are asked in critical appraisal are presented in Table 2.2. Both external validity and internal validity can be compromised due to selection bias. Selection bias is defined as 'Distortions that result from procedures used to select subjects and from factors that influence participation in the study' (Porta and Last 2008). When a study is designed there are a number of populations of interest:

- a target population to which we try to generalize the results

- the source population, the population from which we hope to get the subjects for the study

- eligible population (or intended sample) we identify from which to get the sample

- the actual study population that was recruited.

Table 2.2: Criteria and questions for critical appraisal of studies

Appraisal criterion	Main question	Specific questions for designs
A. Systematic errors		
1. Selection Bias	Was everyone included who should have been included?	Are cases and controls representative of all cases/controls of interest? (CC)
1.1 Volunteer bias	Are participants volunteers?	Exclusion bias is possible in selecting controls (CC)
1.2 Non-response bias	Was the non-response high? Could non-responders be different in any way?	Volunteer bias can occur in cohort studies and cross-sectional studies and in selection of controls (CC)
		Non-response is possible in all designs.
1.3 Loss to follow-up*	Was there loss to follow up?	Follow-up is important in cohort studies (RCS and PCS)
2. Information Bias	Was exposure and outcome clearly defined and accurately measured?	Was there blinding** in measurement of cases and controls (CC)
2.1 Differential misclassification	Do measures truly reflect what they are supposed to measure?	Recall bias is common in all retrospective designs (CC and RCS).
2.2 Non-differential misclassification 2.3 Recall bias	Is exposure or outcome measured using respondent's memory of past events?	Recall bias can occur in CS designs if exposure or outcome are in the past.
B. Random error	Was there a sufficient number of cases selected for investigation? Are power calculations given?	Important for all designs. Estimation more difficult in PCS design as an estimate of incident cases need to be made.
C. Generalizability	How representative are the findings to defined populations?	Was the cohort representative of all with similar exposure? Were respondents representative of the population of interest? (CS and CC)

*Loss to follow-up: in scientific studies participants are followed up from time of recruitment to the end of study. In most studies, a number of participants will leave the study for various reasons. This 'loss to follow-up' can cause bias in the results.

**A blind or blinded experiment is a scientific experiment where some of the persons involved are prevented from knowing certain information that might lead to conscious or subconscious bias on their part, invalidating the results.

CC: Case control study   RCS: Retrospective cohort study

CS: Cross-sectional   PCS: Prospective study

Selection bias occurs when the study population does not represent the target population (see Delgado-Rodriguez and Lorca 2004).

Occurence of NDE: The collective evidence

In Greyson's (1998) review of studies on incidence of NDE it has been noted that there have been a number of errors in past studies, such as:

- bias in the selection of subjects, specifically 'volunteer bias'

- information bias, in studies that have used unreliable measures to classify cases of NDE

- issues of generalizability.

Greyson (1998) argued that by the use of prospective studies, a number of the issues of selection bias can be overcome; however, even prospective studies can have selection bias. Unlike most epidemiological studies of disease, in NDE, the exposure and outcome are not separated by time. The period in which NDE occurs (outcome) is often very short and most studies identify it to be during a period of unconsciousness or death (exposure). Therefore both events happen at the same time.

When one reviews past studies of NDE, there is sufficient evidence that a phenomenon that has been defined as NDE does occur (Moody 1975; Ring 1980). In his review, of studies up to 1998, Greyson (1998) stated that the incidence varies from 0 per cent to 100 per cent but cannot be taken as accurate due to methodological errors. In Table 2.1, we showed more recent studies that show variation in incidence as calculated by the researchers. One of the main factors that may contribute to the variation is that subjects were drawn from population groups (source populations) that had different levels of risk for NDE. Another reason is that some of these studies were not designed for the purpose of estimating incidence (e.g. Corrazza and Schifano 2010).

Critical review of design issues in NDE studies

Selection bias

There are three studies in the review sample, that used a cross-sectional design to estimate the incidence of NDE. Two of them purport to be national samples (Knoblauch, Schmied and Schnettler 2001; Perera,

Padmasekera and Belanti 2005), and the other (Greyson 2003b) a survey of outpatients from a psychiatry department. Knoblauch *et al.*'s study had as one aim to assess 'how many had NDE experiences' (Knoblauch *et al.* 2001 p.20). It is not clear who was selected to answer the questionnaire and volunteer bias is highly likely. In addition, as information on non-response to interviews is not provided, it is difficult to ascertain those who were excluded. Many of these issues are overcome by Perera *et al.* (2005), who used a stratified sample from a national census frame. However, their measure of outcome even though based on the Greyson NDE scale did not use the widely accepted cut-off of more than seven to classify NDE (see p.25). Therefore the incidence may be an overestimate. On the other hand since it was a telephone-based survey it may not estimate the true incidence. Pasricha (2008) in her study usually questioned the head of the household and if they said there was someone with an NDE then they were studied (p.269). This is also an example of bias as the head of household's knowledge of what others experience may not be accurate.

There are four studies that used cohorts of persons with cardiac arrest to study NDE. The first observation to make about these is that the source populations for the studies are different. The main difference was in the inclusion (or exclusion) of persons who had cardiac arrests outside the hospital. For instance in the study in the Netherlands (van Lommel *et al.* 2001), the researchers use both groups, while only those who survived a cardiac arrest outside the hospital were included in the study from Slovenia (Klemenc-Ketis, Kersnik and Grmec 2010). The other studies, only considered cardiac arrest in hospital. The target population used by Greyson (2003a) was cardiac patients, a wider source population than the others, as the objective for the study was different.

Selection bias due to differences from source population to actual study population is seen in Schwaninger *et al.* (2002) who left out those who entered surgical intensive care. Of all possible cardiac arrests that survived in Slovenia, those who were not transferred to hospitals were excluded (Klemenc-Ketis *et al.* 2010). These cases may have been older, younger or less ill than those transferred to hospital. Such information is required to rule out selection bias.

One of the main causes of selection bias in cohort studies is loss to follow-up. In NDE studies this is negligible because the outcome occurs with the exposure. However, non-response bias has to be considered after the cohort is defined. Those who would have had longer periods of unconsciousness may be excluded in the interviews. Unfortunately, in a number of studies information on non-response is not provided. In a study period, those who are unconscious will not be interviewed, and the longer they are unconscious the higher the chance for exclusion. Schwaninger *et al.* (2002) excluded 40 per cent of the study population, which is considered rather high for a study. Schwaninger does not tell us why they were excluded; in general exclusions of over 10 to 15 per cent do not provide a good representation of the study group. In addition information comparing the two groups are not presented to ascertain if selection bias took place. In the study in Slovenia, details of cases of cardiac arrest that were not discharged alive are not provided. All studies of NDE use respondents who had near-death (or clinical death) experiences and survived. For instance in studies using individuals with cardiac arrest, as only those who survive are investigated, the findings from this group only represent the incidence in those who survive a cardiac arrest. An estimate based on those who survive cannot be used to eliminate the incidence of NDE for all those who have a cardiac arrest.

Information bias

Information bias occurs when the measurement of exposure (cardiac arrest) or outcome (NDE) is not clearly defined and objectively measured. Three studies (Parnia *et al.* 2001; van Lommel *et al.* 2001; Klemenc-Ketis *et al.* 2010) measured clinical death, using objective criteria. On the other hand such objective criteria were not used to identify cardiac arrest by Schwaninger *et al.* (2002) and Greyson (2003a). The measurement of outcome in the case of NDE is usually subjective and is prone to misclassification. When we examine the studies included in this review, it is seen that over time researchers have used a tested NDE scale (Greyson 1998). However, in three studies, this scale was not administered to subjects; oral interviews were conducted. In one study the scale was not administered directly to subjects but completed by researchers based on a recorded interview to comply with ethics committee requirements (Schwaninger *et al.* 2002). When more than one interviewer classifies NDE, it is prone to inter-rater (differences between the raters) bias. There is a need to test inter-rater reliability. This has not been reported (Parnia *et al.* 2001; van Lommel *et al.* 2001 and Schwaninger *et al.* 2002).

Amnesia and selective memory are issues in collecting NDE data. In the Netherlands study (van Lommel *et al.* 2001), those who were intubated received high doses of sedatives, which may have affected memory. This may have been the case in other studies too. Older patients with cardiac arrest may remember less about the NDE events, which can account for the higher incidence among younger persons. In general, most of the studies in the series attempted to overcome recall bias by interviewing respondents within a five-day interval.

It is documented in the literature that some persons can have more than one NDE in their lifetime. This poses an issue in calculation of incidence. For instance, in the prospective study in the Netherlands (van Lommel *et al.* 2001) there were 509 successful resuscitations among 344 patients, which can lead to more than one NDE per person. This situation was acknowledged in the previous review of studies of NDE (see Greyson 1998, p.96). This, however, is not the difference between prevalence and incidence, as incidence counts all 'new cases' which in NDE are new episodes of NDE.

Other design issues in NDE studies

The size of the sample is of concern in any study that estimates incidence or is designed to test determinants of NDE. In almost all studies, sample size calculations* and confidence** intervals of the estimates are not provided. These are areas where future studies can make improvements in design and reporting. Furthermore if one were to get information initially from a third party, as evidenced in Pasricha's study (2008) then we have the problem of probable underestimate as well a biased view of a significant other.

Others have recruited persons who have had a close brush with death (Fracasso et al. 2010) as there would be a higher chance of NDE. The subjects in the study by Fracasso *et al.* (2010) were selected from among a small group and were those 'claiming to have memories from a period of unconsciousness associated with a close brush with death ...' (p.265).

In all studies that were conducted with high-risk populations, for example those who have had a cardiac arrest, the results can only be generalized to the specific target population, in this case those who have cardiac arrests.

---

*   Sample size determination is the act of choosing the number of observations to include in a statistical sample. The sample size is an important feature of any empirical study in which the goal is to make inferences about a population from a sample. In practice, the sample size used in a study is determined based on the expense of data collection, and the need to have sufficient statistical power. The latter is calculated by using formulae.

**   Confidence interval is a range of values for a variable of interest, for example a rate constructed so that this range has a specified probability of including the true value of the variable. The specified probability is called the confidence level, and the end points of the confidence interval are called the confidence limits.

Conclusions and future research

A review of recent published studies of NDE was undertaken to assess the evidence on the occurrence of NDE. There are very few population-based studies and the best estimate is from an Australian study that found that approximately 9 per cent of the population has NDE (Perera *et al.* 2005). This is much higher than studies in India (4 per 10,000 population, according to Pasricha 2008). As population studies are very resource intensive, innovative methods are needed to be able to screen for 'likely candidates' before interviews are conducted, a method used by Pasricha (2008) in India but with its own limitations.

More accurate estimates are possible from high-risk populations, but it is important that these estimates cannot be generalized to the general population. Among such high-risk populations, the incidence of NDE is estimated to be between 6 per cent and 23 per cent. However, many of these studies have potential bias. Studies need to be designed in the future to overcome such bias.

The subjective nature of the phenomenon of NDE makes objective measurement difficult. Some questionnaires that have been used will be provided in the phenomenology chapter (Chapter 3). More studies now use Greyson's NDE scale (1983) as the standard. While this trend is useful, it is useful for researchers to collect qualitative data as subjective descriptions can then be compared with different classifications used in other studies. A number of studies have used this technique, but have not carried out tests of reliability for classification, which is one area that future studies can improve on.

The current literature finds that there are more younger persons with NDE. This may be an artifact of selection bias (younger people may be more likely to survive near-death) and recall bias (older people may have loss of memory). New high-risk groups need to be studied for NDE, who may have several advantages, as seen in the study of dialysis patients in Taiwan (Lai *et al.* 2010). Other population groups who are at high risk for NDE may not have yet been studied, such as persons in hospices and those facing end-of-life situations. It may be that collecting data from such groups is complicated given underlying morbidity, such as dementia. On the other hand, these groups are natural cohorts that can be followed up. Therefore we urge future researchers as far as possible to use standardized measures, give details of the questionnaires, etc. and details of the populations studied.

CHAPTER 3

Phenomenology of Near-Death Experiences

KARUPPIAH JAGADHEESAN AND JOHN BELANTI

Personal anecdotes and references to near-death experiences (NDE) have been in existence from time immemorial. However, as outlined in previous chapters, a more detailed systematic exploration of NDE began with the pioneering work of Raymond Moody (1975). Phenomenology is the study of structures of consciousness as experienced from first-person points of view. In this context, phenomenological studies contribute extensively in understanding personal experiences of those who have NDEs. This chapter will focus primarily on clarifying details of such personal experiences. Although phenomenology includes discussion about variations in the manifestation of an experience due to demographic variation, and particularly cultural variations, and other variables, these aspects are not addressed in this chapter, as these issues are covered in subsequent chapters. Nevertheless, it is worth considering the fact that occurrence of NDE has not been correlated with any specific demographic variable (van Lommel 2010).

Phenomenology

A number of features of NDE have been identified. As mentioned in Chapter 1, based on his seminal study, Moody (1975) identified 15 features of NDE. This finding was subsequently validated by Ring (1980). These features could be considered as 'classical features' of NDE. These 15 features are 'ineffability' or difficulty in describing the experience, 'hearing the news' that one has been pronounced dead; feelings of peace and quiet; hearing 'noises' of an unpleasant or pleasant nature; a dark tunnel experience characterized by a sensation of being pulled very rapidly through a dark space of some kind; 'out of the body experience' of seeing one's physical body from a point outside of it; 'meeting others' – having awareness of other beings in one's vicinity; 'encountering and communicating with "the being of light"'; 'the review' – seeing a panoramic review of one's life; a sense of approaching the 'border or limit' crossing of which could lead to non-return; 'coming back' to one's physical body with known purpose or uncertain reason; 'telling others' about the experiences and its importance; the experience having some 'effect on personal lives' in that there is increased appreciation, reflection, intuitiveness and love for others; 'new views of death' characterized by loss of fear; and 'corroboration' – ability to verify things that happened when the physical body was declared dead.

The following vignette, based on the personal experience of one of the authors (John Belanti), depicts the occurrence of this phenomenon in a context of emotional and physical crisis while witnessing a major disaster, which was the tsunami in Thailand in 2004. Before reading this narrative, and for that matter, before going through any individual accounts of NDE, it is worth remembering the cautionary words of Moody (1975). These include his statement that no two accounts of NDE will be identical, no one person will have every single component of the composite experience, persons who were declared 'dead' tend to experience more florid and complete experiences, and those who were 'dead' for a longer period of time go 'deeper' (Moody 1975, p.25).

Narrative 1

I woke up to my bed shaking. Initially I thought it was due to construction next door, so I went back to sleep. I then re-awoke to another stronger shake and realized it was an earthquake when I saw that a bottle on the television was moving. Looking over the balcony from the fourth storey,

I saw that the road along the beach was flooded with water. The room phone then rang advising that there had been an earthquake near by and that we should all evacuate the building and gather on the hill behind the hotel. My brother and I rushed down to get on a scooter to reach a nearby hilltop. I remember that at this point my heart rate was high, and I felt weak, short of breath and had difficulty in thinking.

As we were watching, with our scooter engines on, just about to ride up to the back hill, the ocean water began to recede, quite a long way out. It felt that time had stood still, everyone had frozen, never before had I experienced such a sight. The water then began to return as a thick, fast wave, without breaking, and it got closer and closer. We all fled trying to out-run the water. As we accelerated on the scooters, all I heard was a massive roar like the sound of water behind, and we witnessed another two big waves.

From the hilltop, I experienced a feeling of connectedness with the people around, I remember feeling that 'I' was only a small part of what had just happened and that there were many people who had passed that morning. Around that time, I found myself staring out into the open and experienced calmness and peace. I was in a daydream state, drifting in and out of some vivid thoughts about my own family and certain life experiences, thinking about events of my life and what I have learnt from them. On the second night, emotional and mental exhaustion set in and I recall talking with my brother about how we were happy about what we had done in our lives. We both reflected on shared meaningful events. We then decided to return to our room on the fourth storey accepting death as an option.

For at least two weeks, following the event, after leaving the environment, I experienced a heightened sense of anxiety, and an increased feeling of vulnerability dawned on me again when I watched footage on the television. Once this settled, I began to feel calm again knowing that 'all is just the way it is' and intuitively, I felt the need to trust in that. On returning home, I went through quite a profound psychological and spiritual shift in the way I felt about situations and myself. I initially began to lose interest in certain things and aspects of my behaviour changed, particularly in my responses to perceived frustrating or worrying situations, and I began consciously disengaging from blame and judgemental talk. I also noticed an increase in 'coincidences' as similar situations began emerging that offered opportunity for personal and professional development.

This narrative illustrates that the author (John Belanti) had experienced a few features of NDE as described above (Moody 1975) while facing a critical situation. These features include a sense of peace, life review, telling others and a positive change in life in general.

Major categories of NDEs

Phenomenological analysis of an experience or phenomenon focuses on two aspects – 'form' and 'content'. While 'form' is related to the structural aspects of an experience, 'content' is about the meaning of such experience. As documented, the form of NDE experience is generally characterized by a sense of movement, possibly an out-of-body experience, intense emotions, ineffability, light or darkness, encounter with non-material beings, life-changing messages, and sometimes transcendent elements such as symbols and archetypal images (Bush 2009). As the form of NDE remains fairly uniform, based on the content, these experiences could be grouped into two major categories:

- pleasurable experiences

- distressing experiences.

Pleasurable NDEs

In general, NDEs are considered pleasant and positively transforming and this is evidenced by the fact that the current literature has higher reporting of pleasurable than unpleasant experiences (Bush 2009). In this context, the above findings of Moody (1975), that give no evidence of distressing experiences (Greyson and Bush 1992), except 'noises' of an unpleasant nature (in some), could be considered to illustrate features of the pleasurable type.

Distressing NDEs

Greyson and Bush (1992) have described three subtypes of distressing NDE. These include:

1. prototypical NDEs interpreted as terrifying

2. experience of non-existence or eternal void

3. experiences with hellish imagery.

In the first type, prototypical features such as a bright light, a tunnel, etc. are interpreted is terrifying and often, loss of ego control is the terrifying aspect of the experience. The second type is characterized by a paradoxical sensation of ceasing to exist entirely or being condemned to a featureless void for eternity. It is also associated with sense of despair about life. This type tends to have only fewer elements of prototypical features and does not appear to change to the pleasant type with time. The third type includes hellish symbolism, such as demons or falling into a dark pit, and it tends to have only few aspects of prototypical features. This type remains stable with time. Later, Rommer (2000) reported a fourth type characterized by life review with external judgement.

Based on the literature review, Bush (2009) reports that distressing NDE occur in both life-threatening and non-life-threatening experiences and that there is under-reporting due to fear, shame, social stigma, and to avoid burdening others and reliving the experience. Further, this author suggests that distressing experiences represent the depths/intensity of spiritual experience and may produce a long-lasting emotional and psycho-spiritual trauma, and there is no evidence that these experiences are punishment for faults in one's beliefs or behaviours.

Typology

A few investigators categorized NDE into subtypes. Michael Sabom (1982) reviewed 71 incidents of NDE and suggested three types – autoscopic (30%), transcendental (54%) and mixed type (17%) with features of both types.

Greyson (1985) examined subtypes of NDE through cluster analysis of 89 NDEs that were measured through the Near-Death Experience Scale and reported three subtypes – transcendental (42.7%), affective (41.6%) and cognitive (15.7%). These types did not correlate with demographic features and with specific cause of near-death event. Nonetheless, there was a significant finding that the cognitive type occurred rarely when death was anticipated (e.g. suicide attempts, exacerbation of chronic illness or complications of surgery), whereas all three types occurred with equal frequency in sudden and unanticipated near-death events (e.g. accidents, cardiac arrests or anaphylactic reactions).

Atwater (2007) proposed four subtypes – initial experience (or non-experience or awakening), unpleasant (or hell-like or distressing), pleasant (or heaven-like or radiant) and transcendental (or collective universality).

The first type (76% of children and of 20% of adults) is characterized by limited number of experiences (1–3 elements) and experiences such as loving nothingness, the living dark, a friendly voice, a brief out-of-body experience, or a manifestation of some type. The second type (3% of children and 15% of adults) include encounter with a threatening void, stark limbo, hellish purgatory, scenes of a startling and unexpected indifference (like being shunned), hauntings from one's past, life reviews and some previews. The third type (19% of children and 47% of adults) includes loving family unions, reassuring religious figures, or light beings, validation that life counts, affirmative and inspiring dialogue, life reviews and some previews. The last type (2% of children and 18% of adults) is related to exposure to other-worldly dimensions and scenes beyond the individual's frame of reference, and sometimes includes revelations of greater truths.

Progression (Staging)

Moody (1975) suggested that NDEs progress in such a way that initial experiences (e.g. ineffability) occur more commonly than the later experiences (e.g. reaching a border or limit). Kenneth Ring (1980) carried out a systematic study to verify Moody's findings and reported that progression of NDE happens in stages with each stage being characterized by certain experiences. Accordingly, there are five stages. Stage 1 was affective in nature with feelings of peace and well-being, and this was reported in 60 per cent of the participants. In Stage 2 (37%), there was body separation (out-of-body experience), increased acuity of mental and perceptual process, sense of movement of body in non-physical realm and mindset of 'observer-like detachment'. Stage 3 (23%) was characterized by entering the darkness, Stage 4 (16%) by seeing the light, and Stage 5 (10%) by entering the light with the experience of entering into another world, brilliant visual and auditory experiences, and meeting deceased relatives.

After-effects

While some of Moody's elements – telling others, effects on lives and new views on death – are related to after-effects of NDE, the first systematic effort in exploring after-effects was begun by Ring (1980). Subsequently, a number of other investigators have explored after-effects (van Lommel 2010). Ring (1980) categorized after-effects into three major areas:

1. personality and value changes

2. attitudes towards religion

3. attitude towards death.

This research showed that following NDE, people showed changes in their personality and values; they reported increased appreciation of life, personal renewal and the search for purpose in life. Positive personality changes were usually characterized by increased self-esteem and increased love, compassion, empathy, tolerance and understanding towards others. Regarding religion, people reported increased religiosity in the form of inner religious impulse and prayer, appreciation of God and religious tolerance but fewer formal rituals. There was no change in belief in God and there was increased belief in life after death. A significant observation was that people had reported significant reduction in or no fear towards death following NDE. Van Lommel (2010) has reviewed the literature on this topic and the findings of this review are summarized as follows. The observed changes are improved self-worth and positive change in self-image, increased compassion for others, enhanced appreciation of life with a purpose or goal, reduced or absence of fear of death, a belief in life after death, a decline in religious affiliation, increased religious sentiment, physical changes (e.g. heightened sensitivity, ability to direct healing power), enhanced intuition, and psychological difficulties due to change in attitude towards roles, relationships and conventions, and due to societal expectations.

The following narrative highlights the negative after-effects, particularly the role of societal attitude in contributing to such difficulties.

Narrative 2

Mr A is a 54-year-old man who was admitted to a residential rehabilitation programme for psychiatric rehabilitation with a background of chronic depression, lack of family support and difficult childhood experiences. He had two transient ischaemic attacks in the past. He had abused cannabis and alcohol many years ago and had been prescribed an antidepressant.

He narrated an experience which he had while he was undergoing an angiogram to evaluate his cerebral vascular pattern. He reported that his experience was characterized by the appearance of a white light and movement of his body to a higher location from where he could see what was going on around him. He said he had an amazing feeling of peace and he could hear the conversation of staff. After a brief period, he returned to his body and while doing so, he felt terribly sad. He denied hearing any sounds or having any additional visual experiences at that time. After recovery from this episode, he said he started to feel sad, as he wanted to stay up there, and later, he shared his experience with staff.

He stated that his experience was declared as an adverse reaction to the procedure. As a result, he felt he was not understood and supported given that he had had an extraordinary experience that was meaningful for him. Around that time, he was started on antidepressants, which he continued to take for many years. He also mentioned that he felt less supported by his family and friends, as many of them did not believe such an experience could occur and so he stopped talking about it. He reported loss of interest in his hobbies and preferred activities following this experience. Upon questioning, he reported that health professionals could have allowed him to talk about this experience in the beginning. He reported that he has always felt he was not happy to return to this life after that experience.

Diagnostic clarification

There are a number of conditions that need to be differentiated from NDEs.

Altered states of pathological nature

Psychopathological states are worth discussing in this context and these include depersonalization, derealization and dissociation. Noyes and Kletti (1976) observed that individuals develop depersonalization when faced with life-threatening danger and this phenomenon is characterized by certain features, including review and transcendence. These authors proposed that depersonalization suggested an adaptive response of human biological and psychological substrates under dangerous situations. This proposition is challenged by the current nosological understanding of depersonalization. According to the *Diagnostic and Statistical Manual of Mental Disorders, Fourth Edition, Text Revision (DSM-IV-TR)*, depersonalization is a feeling of being detached from, and being an outside observer of, one's mental processes or body (e.g. feeling like one is in a dream) (American Psychiatric Association 2000). Whereas, in *The ICD-10 Classification of Mental and Behavioural Disorders Tenth Revision (ICD-10)*, depersonalization is characterized by feeling that one's own feelings and/or experiences are detached, distant, not one's own, lost and so on. *ICD-10* describes derealization as objects, people and/or surroundings seeming unreal, distant, artificial, colourless, lifeless, and so on (Word Health Organization 1992).

Another phenomenon that needs to be differentiated from NDE is dissociation. According to *DSM-IV TR* (American Psychiatric Association 2000), dissociation is disruption of the usually integrated functions of consciousness, memory, identity, or perception of the environment. However, there are two other approaches that are being used for the purpose of research in this area. According to the narrower approach dissociation is division of consciousness or personality whereas the broader approach conceptualizes dissociation as breakdown of integrated functions (Isaac and Chand 2006).

A common factor amongst all these experiences is that they occur when an individual is faced with anxiety-provoking situations. These conditions could occur as one-off or recurring in nature, as, for example, with depersonalization disorder (Reutens, Nielsen and Sachdev 2010). It is important to note that all these experiences are known to occur as part of depression, anxiety disorders (depersonalization disorder, dissociative disorders, etc.), and other psychiatric conditions (Reutens *et al.* 2010). In general, when these experiences occur, an individual is distressed and there is a negative effect on their overall functioning. NDE could be differentiated from these experiences by the fact that such experiences occur close to the time of death, when often there is no time for the individual to process the situation as threatening and so the usual emotional experience is a sense of peace, joy and bliss. Further, NDE often leads to a positive impact on one's life (van Lommel 2010).

Hallucinations

These are perceptions that occur without any discernible external stimuli and such experience could involve any sensory modality, so they can be auditory, visual, etc. Two phenomena that need discussion are autoscopic hallucination and multimodal hallucinations. In autoscopic hallucination, a subject can see their own body in front at a certain distance. This image can be transparent, or coloured and definite, or show expressive movements. This phenomenon can occur in cerebral disease and psychiatric conditions (e.g. depression, schizophrenia). This experience is almost always recognized as a pathological event and the emotional reaction may be anxiety or surprise depending upon the mental state (Lishman 1998). In contrast to independently occurring hallucinations, multimodal hallucinations are characterized by the occurrence of hallucinations of different modalities occurring at the same time. Such complex experiences could lead to vivid visual and somatic experiences. It is important to note that these experiences are distressing to the individuals, that they are often recurring in nature, that there is co-existence of other psychopathology and that they occur in the context of psychiatric and neurological conditions (Chesterman and Boast 1994). In addition to the situational criteria, other features such as onset, progression and after-effects differentiate NDE from these psychopathological phenomena.

Drug-induced states

Anaesthetic agents (e.g. ketamine), endorphins, psychedelic drugs (e.g. Lysergic acid diethylamide (LSD), Dimethyltryptamine (DMT), etc.) are known to cause NDE-like experiences (Bates and Stanley 1985; van Lommel 2010). These drug-induced experiences are observed to be less complex when compared with that of NDE (Bates and Stanley 1985). Nonetheless, there is a theoretical proposition that DMT, which is endogenously produced, could play a role in the experience of enhanced consciousness in near-death experience (van Lommel 2010).

Out-of-body experiences (OBE)

This experience is characterized by movement in the centre of awareness wherein an individual can see the world from a location outside their body. An OBE can occur by itself or as part of NDE. When it occurs as part of NDE, usually other features of NDE occur along with OBE. Gabbard, Twemlow and Jones (1981) reported that only 10 per cent of 339 subjects reported occurrence of OBE in near-death states. On comparing the phenomenology of OBE and NDE, Gabbard *et al.* observed that persons with NDE are more likely to experience hearing noises at the early stage of experience, tunnel experience, seeing their physical body from a distance, and being able to sense other beings in non-physical form, particularly deceased people of emotional significance. They report that feelings of peace and serenity are common to both experiences. According to them, proximity to death seems to provide certain characteristic features, which differentiate NDE from other similar experiences.

Epilepsy and organic states, including brain stimulation

Temporal lobe epilepsy (TLE) needs to be discussed specifically. Because of location and connection with other cerebral structures, abnormality in temporal lobes can lead to epileptic phenomena that can manifest as complex visual and somatic experiences, including mystical experience. A review reports that 0.4–3.1 per cent of patients with partial epilepsy had religious experiences during seizures (ictal phase) and 3.9 per cent had religious premonitory symptoms or auras. About 1.3 per cent of all epilepsy patients and 2.2 per cent of TLE patients reported religious experience immediately following seizure (postictal phase) (Devinsky and Lai 2008). One of the theories of NDE is related to the possible role of temporal lobe. However, there is no substantial evidence to prove that there is a temporal pathology in all NDEs and absence of brain activity recorded at the time of NDE suggests that these phenomena could not be explained by temporal lobe pathology (van Lommel 2010). Further, organic conditions such as epilepsy tend to manifest with other clinical features such as dysfunction, cognitive deficits and psychopathology (Lishman 1998). Blanke et al. (2004), based on a small study involving neurological patients, suggested that OBE and autoscopy are due to a failure of neuronal mechanisms necessary for the integrity of sense of personal space and the integrity between personal and extra-personal space. Although it is an interesting observation, it will be difficult to generalize this finding to all NDE. As discussed above, NDE could be differentiated from these (organic) experiences based on its phenomenology, onset at the proximity to death (physical and psychological) and course.

Meditation and cosmic consciousness

Bates and Stanley (1985) discuss this topic and state that NDE could be differentiated from meditation (transcendental meditation) wherein the subject moves towards pure consciousness and that near-death-like experiences are considered part of the healing process of meditation. These authors also describe cosmic consciousness as permanent, simultaneous perception of pure awareness of the external world. According to them, NDE and cosmic consciousness have a similar form. Subjects in either state report a sense of unity with the world, timelessness, increased perceptual acuity and lucid thinking. On the other hand, the content of these experiences such as communicating with a being of light or travelling in dark tunnels are not reported in the literature on transcendental meditation.

Instruments for evaluation of NDE
Weighted Core Experience Index (WCEI) Scale

As outlined in Chapter 2, perhaps the first NDE ratings scale was that of Ring (1980). The items were selected based on a literature search. This instrument has a structured interview schedule and a rating scale (see Appendices 1 and 2). A major aspect of the interview schedule is about gathering information about elements of NDEs and information about religious beliefs and practices. The Tape rating form (Appendix 2) is to be used after completion of tape recording of the interview (Appendix 1). The rating form has some blank entries so that new experiences not mentioned in the form could be noted. Items have been rated on a five-point scale and there are ten items that have weighted scoring. These items include:

1. subjective sense of being dead

2. feelings of peace, painlessness, pleasantness, etc.

3. sense of bodily separation

4. sense of entering a dark region

5. entering a presence/hearing a voice

6. taking stock of one's life

7. seeing or being enveloped in light

8. seeing beautiful colours

9. entering into light

10. encountering visible spirits.

Based on the total score, the depth of an individual's experience could be categorized as follows: not a core experiencer (score < 6), moderate experiencer (score = 6–9) and deep experiencer (score > 10). This scale has been used in research (e.g. van Lommel *et al.* 2001). However, this scale needs validation on certain psychometric properties (Greyson 1983).

Near-Death Experience Scale

This is a 16-item scale with each item scored from zero to two (Appendix 3). A cut-off score of seven and above was considered to indicate presence of NDE (Greyson 1983). The items are grouped into 4 factors – cognitive, affective, paranormal and transcendental. The cognitive domain includes four items – time distortion, thought acceleration, life review and sudden understanding. The affective domain includes four items – peace, joy, feeling of cosmic unity and light. Four items of paranormal experiences include sensory vividness, extrasensory perception, precognitive visions and OBE. The transcendental domain includes four items – unfamiliar environment, unidentified presence, religious or deceased spirits, and border or point of no return. The scale has been reported to have good reliability and validity measures (Greyson 1983). Subsequently, the first item about time distortion was modified to include both 'speeding up' and 'slowing down'. In addition, a cut-off (five or more) for each subscale was introduced so that a dominant pattern or theme of NDE could be identified. According to this scoring, an NDE will be considered to be 'cognitive NDE' with a score of five or more on the cognitive domain, irrespective of the scores in other domains. Likewise, 'transcendental NDE' is indicated with a score of five or more on this domain but less than five in the cognitive domain. 'Affective NDE' will have a score of five or more on the affective domain but less than five on cognitive and transcendental domains. 'Paranormal NDE' will be indicated with a score of five or more on this domain but with a score of below five in other subscales (Greyson 1990). Lange, Greyson and Houran (2004) applied Rasch model[*] on NDE scale to verify existence of a hierarchical structure or relationship among features of NDE. In this study, analysis of those who were classified as True NDErs (those claimed to have had an NDE and had a raw score of at least seven on NDE scale)

---

[*]   Rasch model examines the relationship between the probability of being observed in a particular category, and the difference between an individual's ability and an item's difficulty – for further information refer to www.rasch.org.

confirmed that there was a probabilistic progression of features of NDE. In a follow-up study, the NDE Scale was administered to the available participants from the original cohort (63%) and was found to produce similar results without any change in score for the four factors and 16 items (Greyson 2007).

NDE Questionnaire

This questionnaire was used in the Australian National Survey for NDEs (Perera, Padmasekara and Belanti 2005). The items were derived from the NDES (Greyson 1983) but only items that tended to occur with high frequency were included. These selected items were modified to suit telephone survey. This questionnaire included four questions, with additional prompts as necessary (see Appendix 4):

1. At any time in your life have you ever felt that you were close to the point of dying?

2. Can you briefly describe the situation that you were in when this happened?

3. What, if anything, did you see or hear or feel during this NDE? What else? Anything else?

4. In that near-death situation did any of the following things happen? (Prompts given in Appendix 4)

Conclusion

In phenomenological terms, NDE is characterized by a set of clearly distinguishable features. Although no one element is universal in its occurrence (Moody 1975), certain features tend to occur commonly. These 'signature features' are OBE, a light that shines brighter than the sun, a 'voice-less' voice that speaks telepathically, a calming feeling of total acceptance and unconditional love, a sudden knowingness and feeling the need or being told to return (Atwater 2007).

The structural aspects of this phenomenon remain fairly stable whereas the meaning and the degree of expression or unfolding (or depth) of this experience vary. In general, NDEs are pleasant, and life transforming. Nonetheless, a small proportion of experiences are unpleasant and distressing.

A number of psychiatric and organic states could resemble or present with some features of NDE. Likewise, certain spiritual experiences could include near-death-like experiences. Clinicians need to be aware of these conditions. A carefully applied phenomenological approach will help in differentiating these experiences from NDE.

The available instruments or scales vary in their degree of structure and the amount of time needed for administration. While the well-structured WCEI and the survey-focused NDE Questionnaire will be highly applicable in research settings, the NDE Scale has scope for use in both clinical and research settings.

CHAPTER 4

Dealing with Diversity

Cross-Cultural Aspects of Near-Death Experiences

ORNELLA CORAZZA AND K.A.L.A. KURUPPUARACHCHI

Introduction

Individuals have their own idiosyncratic ways of being. In group situations these may become modified. The combined influence of learning, language, religion, socio-political and cultural dimensions colours human attitudes toward death and life to an indefinite degree. National surveys and some studies on near-death experiences (NDEs) mainly from Western European countries have been summarized in Chapter 2. Non-Western NDEs have been comprehensively reviewed by Kellehear (2008). He cites studies from China, India, Thailand and Tibet (the Asian subcontinent), West New Britain, a province of Papua New Guinea on the island of New Britain, Guam and New Zealand Maoris (the Pacific area) and from Native American, African and Australian hunter-gatherer communities. He eloquently argued that 'There is an important need to link the cultural, psychological, and physiological data to appreciate the interrelationship between the three experiential domains in generating a complete and balanced portrait of human experiences near death' (Kellehear 2008, p.250). The field of NDE is replete with descriptions in the English language of NDE phenomena mainly from the 'Westerners' eyes. In this chapter the authors will explore NDEs from different countries and draw on their own experience to explore the commonalities and variations of NDEs in the countries mentioned.

Reports of NDE

China

We know relatively little about NDE in China. The most popular work has been carried out by Carl Becker of the University of Kyoto (Becker 1981). He made a study of three traditional monks, who were exponents of the foundation of the Pure Land Buddhism. Each one of the three monks reported a period of illness, during which they all experienced either an NDE or a death-bed vision (DBV), while still reasonably unconscious. During these accounts neither tunnel experience nor out-of-body experience was reported.

More recently, another study was carried out by Zhi-ying and Jian-Xun in 1987. The authors looked at the accounts of 81 survivors of the 1976 Tangshan earthquake in China. Among these, 72 reported an experience similar to an NDE (Zhi-ying and Jian-Xun 1992). The most distinctive features were: 'sensations of the world being exterminated, a sense of weightlessness, a feeling of being pulled or squeezed' as well as the most common 'feeling estranged from the body, unusually vivid thoughts, loss of emotions, unusual bodily sensations, life seeming like a dream, a feeling of dying, a feeling of peace or euphoria, a life review or "panoramic memory", and thinking unusually fast' (Zhi-ying and Jian-Xun 1992, p.46).

Japan

It would appear that the published literature on NDEs is sparse. Yamamura (1998) studied NDEs in a group of 48 consecutive patients. Thirty seven per cent reported NDEs. Among the NDE reported there were such elements as flying in a dark void space with dim light ahead, encountering dead relatives or friends, standing at the boundary of a brook, river or pond, and returning to the world in response to a voice calling from behind. Perhaps the largest study in the country has been carried out by Takashi Tachibana. He is an esteemed journalist in the country, who made a popular survey of four hundred individuals who had survived in life-threatening circumstances. In his work entitled *Near-Death Experience* (1994), which is quite popular in Japan, he argues that the most common features of a Japanese NDE are the visions of long, dark rivers and beautiful flowers. Of greater academic relevance are probably the research results of another NDE investigation carried out by Yoshia Hata and his research team at the University of Kyorin (Hata *et al.* in Hadfield 1991). Researchers interviewed 17 patients, who recovered from a situation where there had been minimal signs of life. Most of them had suffered heart attacks, asthma attacks, or drug poisoning. Eight of them reported memories during unconsciousness (47%). Nine had no memories at all (53%). Of the eight who had an experience, clear visions of rivers or ponds largely prevailed. Such elements have also been emphasized in Takashi Tachibana's popular survey.

One of the most interesting findings of Hata's study is that five of the eight participants (62.5%) reported negative experiences, dominated by fear, pain or suffering. So it was for a 73-year-old lady, who had an NDE as a consequence of a cardiac arrest. She said: 'I saw a cloud filled with dead people. It was a dark, gloomy day. I was chanting sutras. I believed they could be saved if they chanted sutras, so that is what I was telling them to do' (Hadfield 1991, p.11). Negative NDEs seem not to be that common in Western accounts, although as Peter and Elizabeth Fenwick observed, they are probably under-reported because they are less likely to be communicated to others than positive experiences (Fenwick and Fenwick 1995).

Another small case study was carried out at the *Centre of Death and Life Studies* at the University of Tokyo, among three Japanese who survived a life-threatening circumstance (Corazza 2008). One of these was a 66-year-old Tai Chi Master, who had a very powerful NDE, which changed her life. Sixteen years before the interview, she was very sick. She lost consciousness and was resuscitated in the emergency care unit of a hospital in Tokyo. The doctor told her later that her heart had stopped beating for a while and that she was considered clinically dead for an unknown period of time (she couldn't remember). She described having a vision of a river, which separated her side from that of the Realm of Dead (or 'Yomi'). She said: 'As I got closer, at the very end of the other side of the river, I saw my mother who passed away 18 years ago. I could see only her face because a group of children monks, dressed in white and black, masked the rest of her body. The children were very noisy. I moved closer, to see my mother. She looked very worried and she said: "Don't come here! Go back!" So I turned back and regained consciousness in the hospital. At that very moment, I heard a nurse calling my name' (Corazza 2008, p.60).

India

More evidence emerged from several studies which were carried out in India. One of these was carried out by Satwant Pasricha and Ian Stevenson (Pasricha and Stevenson 1986). This was based on 16 individuals with NDEs in India. The authors observed that experiences were characterized by the meeting with Yamraj, the king of the dead, or his messengers, called Yamdoots, or 'the man with the book', Chitragupta. Curiously, near-death experiencers (NDErs) were often 'sent back' to life because of a mistake in the identity of the person. An example quoted in their study is that of Mr Vasudev Pandey, who was interviewed in 1975. This person was considered dead and taken to a cremation ground. At this time, some signs of life aroused the attention of those present and Mr Vasudev was removed to the hospital where doctors tried to bring him back to life. He remained unconscious for three days. When he regained consciousness, he told the following story to those who were present: 'Two persons caught me and took me with them. I felt tired after walking some distance; they started to drag me. My feet became useless. Then there was a man setting up. He looked dreadful and was all black. He was wearing no clothes. He said in a rage [to the attendants who had brought Vasudev] "I had asked you to bring Vasudev the gardener. Our garden is drying up. You have brought Vasudev the student" (Pasricha and Stevenson 1986, p.166). Mr Vasudev's gardener, who was present when Mr Vasudev narrated his NDE, died the following day.

Once again the content of Indian NDE differs from those reported in Western societies where NDErs are not usually able to give a reason for their recovery and if they do so, they are more likely to say that they were 'sent back' because deceased relatives or friends told them that their 'time has not yet come'. A different interpretation of the phenomenon has been given by Susan Blackmore who placed an advertisement in *The Times* of India on 2 November 1991 in order to find potential Indian

NDErs. Although she had 19 replies, she was able to interview only nine of them. Her findings are quite dissimilar from those reported in Pasricha and Stevenson's study where 38 per cent of respondents described a tunnel experience. This evidence supports her theories that there is a biological explanation of the phenomenon (Blackmore 1993).

Another study was carried out in India by Osis and Haraldsson in order to determine the extent of cultural variations in death-bed visions (DBVs). A similar investigation was carried out in the US. They published their results in a book called *At the Hour of Death* (Osis and Haraldsson 1977), which discusses a large number of cultural variations. One of these regards the vision of beings of light, or religious figure, during the experience. The identity of the religious figure (in the vision) was also quite a problem in adult cases. If a patient sees a radiant man clad in white who induces in him an inexplicable experience of harmony and peace, he might interpret the apparition in various ways: as an angel, Jesus, or God; or if he is a Hindu, Krishna, Shiva, or Deva (Osis and Haraldsson, 1977 p.37).

Although one might think that the interpretation given varies according to the religious backgrounds, the authors commented that this did not 'significantly affect the purpose' of the figure seen, and the sight of a dead or a religious figure was 'surprisingly similar on both sides of the globe – 78 per cent for the United States and 77 per cent for India' (Osis and Haraldsson 1977, pp.90–91). An important question about this study is whether these visions were the result of the administration of a particular drug, or whether these were real visions. The answer is that the consciousness of over 60 per cent of the people was absolutely clear and no form of sedative was administered (Osis and Haraldsson 1977, p.70). Only in 30 per cent of the cases it was moderately impaired. Although Osis and Haraldsson's research relates primarily to the phenomenology of death-bed visions, which are defined as occurring in the 24 hours before dying, rather than NDEs, the study presents a considerable amount of data able to reinforce later studies into the phenomenology of NDEs.

Another more recent case report that took place during a surgical procedure featured NDE characteristics, such as memories of travelling in dark terrain, travelling in the dark towards some bright light, remembering people whispering that she is dead (Panditrao, Singh and Panditrao 2010).

Sri Lanka

There are many anecdotal reports and a couple of books have been published on NDEs in the Sinahala language. Jayawardana (2007) published over 20 cases of NDE, along with other related phenomena. A study involving suicide attempters found that none had an NDE, although some of those questioned reported an awareness of the phenomena (Kuruppuarachchi *et al.* 2008). In another ongoing study, over 800 patients admitted to a teaching hospital have been questioned. Approximately 20 per cent among those who had come close to dying reported NDE. It is remarkable that a similar proportion was reported in the Dutch prospective study of cardiac arrest patients (van Lommel *et al.* 2001).

In order to understand the diversity as well as common features of NDEs illustrative case histories are presented.

A 42-year-old female of the Islamic faith experienced NDE after a massive amount of blood loss following a miscarriage. She mentioned that she felt as if her thoughts were moving very fast and she recalled all pleasant events in her life in a second. She claimed that she was floating among the clouds and suddenly saw a dazzling bright light. She also described that her feelings were very intense and strong. She felt that she could understand anything about science and about the world. She also mentioned that she remembered a male voice calling her.

A 50-year-old Sinhala Christian male presented with NDE following a myocardial infarction. He was out of his body and he described that thoughts were moving very rapidly. He also said that he understood many things that he previously never realized and felt a great sense of calm. He observed a very bright light. He also saw his dead father wearing white clothes. He did not want to come back and felt he was sent back by someone. He also experienced out-of-body experience.

A Sinhala Buddhist 38-year-old female became unconscious during an episode of Dengue Haemorrhagic Fever. After recovery she described her experiences during the 'unconscious period' vividly. She described how her thought content increased and her thoughts were moving very fast. She felt calm and felt as if she could understand many things about the world and herself. She too described seeing a bright light. She claimed that she had seen her dead father and had experienced the sense of out-of-body experience. She experienced the 'oneness' of the entire world as she felt that the entire world is in unison. She mentioned that it was an extremely pleasant experience for her.

A married Sinhala Buddhist, a retired professional man in his 70s had developed a cardiac arrest during prostatectomy and was successfully resuscitated within a couple of minutes. He explained his experience subsequently, that he got detached from his body and floated in the air and then wandered towards the village temple and worshipped a sacred Bo tree (*Ficus religiosa*). It was a very pleasant experience for him. He mentioned that he felt extremely unhappy after realizing that he had come back to his body. He became depressed and subsequently committed suicide.

A cardiologist reported NDE in one of her patients. The patient was a Sinhala Buddhist priest who had a cardiac arrest and was subsequently successfully resuscitated. It is reported that he remembered leaving his physical body and starting to float in space. He also recalled meeting with 'deities' well known in the Sri Lankan culture, and meeting with beautiful angels and communicating with them. It was a very pleasant experience for him and he wished to re-experience it.

Traditionally Sri Lankan families are closely knit and 'transgenerational learning' particularly with regard to the religious beliefs and customs plays a major role in shaping the views and belief systems of the people in Sri Lanka. The majority (about 70%) are Sinhala Buddhists. Buddhism has a significant impact on the Sinhala culture (Wickramasinghe 2006a). Sri Lankans generally follow the Theravada or Hinayana school of Buddhism which is regarded as the original orthodox Buddhism whereas countries like China, Japan, Tibet follow the Mahayana school which is a form of Buddhism of later development. Buddhism emphasizes the doctrine of 'No Soul or No Self' (*Anatta*) (Rahula 2006). For self-preservation man has created the idea of soul. According to Buddhism even after the physical body has ceased to function the energies continue to take another shape or form which is called another life and there is continuance in the world cycle which is known as Samsara and one will be born again and again and the fruits of one's actions (karma) are carried over to the next birth or subsequent births. The ultimate goal of Buddhism is to attain enlightenment or 'Nirvana' to end the rebirth and suffering. Therefore the concept of rebirth is a central dogma of the Sinhala culture. Although Buddhism as preached by the Buddha did not advocate blind faith (Wickramasinghe 2006b), religious beliefs especially from Hindu traditions have invaded the psyche of the average practising Buddhist. Sri Lankan culture, their attitudes and belief systems are also influenced by the European ethos due to invasions over the centuries. Research and writings on NDE is sparse in the Sri Lankan literature, but death-bed visions are more commonly acknowledged. This is exemplified by the experiences at the time of the death of a renowned ancient Sri Lankan king Dutugemunu (*Dutthagamini*) who ruled Sri Lanka several centuries ago. He is said to have seen six deities in chariots calling from six different heavens in order to accompany him to a heaven in a chariot (Bullis 2005). Well-researched case histories of rebirth in Sri Lanka have been documented (Story 2000) and it is of interest to note that children who speak about their previous lives have been found in all major religious communities in Sri Lanka (Haraldsson 2001).

Case histories seen in Sri Lanka show that many have had NDE similar to NDE encountered among Western people such as seeing bright light, meeting dead relatives, similar out-of-body experiences, feeling peace, etc. The phenomena have been observed not only among the majority Buddhists but also amongst the people with other religions such as Muslims and Christians. Most of the people mentioned that it was a pleasant experience, and some with cardiac arrests claimed that they observed the resuscitation procedure. The majority of them described the experience vividly. As has been said, many had experiences similar to experiences of the other parts of the world, particularly that of the West, including floating and lack of desire to return to the body. Also some reported a culturally coloured description such as going to the temple and meeting religious figures. Fearful experiences (while seeing sinful acts done in the earlier age of life) in a case with NDE have been documented (Jayawardana 2007).

Melanesia

Dorothy A. Counts reported three cases of NDE among the population of Kalilai, in the province of Western New Britain, known as Melanesia. From these accounts emerged a vision of the after-life characterized by factories and wage employment (Counts 1983). For instance, a person she interviewed found himself walking through a field of flowers to a road that forked in two. In each fork of the road a man was standing persuading the NDEr to come with him. The NDEr picked one of the forks at random:

> The man took my hand and we entered a village. There we found a long ladder that led up into a house. We climbed the ladder but when we got to the top I heard a voice saying: 'It

isn't time for you to go home. Stay there. I'll send a group of people to take you back [...]. So they took me back down the steps. I wanted to go back to the house, but I couldn't because it turned and I realized that it was not on posts. It was just hanging there in the air, turning around as if it were on an axel (*sic*). If I wanted to go to the door, the house would turn and there would be another part of the house where I was standing. There were all kinds of things inside this house, and I wanted to see them all. There were men working with steel, and some men building ships, and another group of men building cars. I was standing staring when this man said: 'It's not time for you to be here. Your time is yet to come. I'll send some people to take you back...you must go back.' I was to go back, but there was no road for me to follow, so the voice said: 'Let him go down.' Then there was a beam of light and I walked along it. I walked down the steps, and then when I turned to look there was nothing but forest... So I walked along the beam of light, through the forest and along a narrow path. I came back to my house and re-entered my body and I was alive again. (Counts 1983, pp.199–120)

According to Counts this 'unusual' kind of NDE vision relates to Kaliais' beliefs that the after-life is characterized by 'divinely given technologies, including factories, automobiles, highways, airplanes, European houses and buildings in great numbers, and manufactured goods' (Counts 1983, p.130). She also observed how the content of the paradise varies and seems to be culturally defined: 'North Americans and Europeans see beautiful gardens, while Kaliai find an industrialized world of factories, highways, and urban sprawl [...].' The culturally structured nature of these experiences is consistent with the explanation that out-of-the body and NDE are the result of a psychological state known as hypnagogic sleep. The Kaliai data presented here suggest that this, rather than an objectively experienced 'life after death' is the most reasonable explanation for the phenomenon (Counts 1983, pp.132–133).

Other substantial differences between Melanesian NDE and those reported in Western countries arise from her study. There was no claim of viewing the body or possessing a new one, nor was there any report of floating sensations or feeling exhilarated with the usual feelings of joy and peace. Auditory sensations were absent and most noticeable were the description of a 'journey' along a road or path. No experiencer recalled moving through a tunnel. Only one of them claimed to have met a personage 'dressed in white' (Counts 1983). Against these differences, the anthropologist was able to identify few similarities. She observes: 'experiencers regretted leaving the place in which they had found themselves, and they also reported encountering others, including some who had died at an earlier time' (Counts 1983, pp.131–132).

Summary of comparison of non-Western and Western NDEs

The people with NDE who could be interviewed after a while mentioned that they have widened the perspectives of the life. Some of them seem to have become more religious and generous following the experience, thus confirming the universality not only of the experience but also of its after-effects. Culture too has an impact on NDE although not consistently. For example, it has been shown that an Indian person is more likely to see Yama, the King of Death, or his messengers called *Yamdoots* (Pasricha and Stevenson 1986), rather than Christ or Madonna. On the contrary, others, like Cherie Sutherland, have reported cases where the content of the experience was actually different from the cultural or religious background of the person who reported the experience (Sutherland 1995).

The idea that NDEs are identical in different countries is particularly appealing to those who support a narrowly biological explanation of the phenomenon. There are various physiological, psychological or neurophysiological explanations of the dying brain and the psychological interpretations which may be elicited in the dying person (e.g. Blackmore 1982; Blackmore and Troscianko 1988; Carr 1982; Sotelo *et al.* 1985). A more in-depth discussion of the pathophysiology is presented in Chapter 6.

Eastern traditions have grasped the esoteric concepts in various ways. For example, we find the idea of *Purusa* in Yoga, *Atman* in Vedanta, *Tao* in Taoism, which all refer to the field, which is called 'authentic self' (Nishida 1990). Even more interestingly, in Tibetan tradition, there is a phenomenon called *delok*, which literally means 'returned from the dead'. The name *deloks* is given to people who seemingly 'die' as a result of an illness, and find themselves travelling in the *Bardo*, before returning to life again (Rinpoche 1992). A concept among certain Buddhists is that there is an Astral body and a state of Interim Existence that prevails between death and rebirth (Rewathe-Thero and Wijethilake 2001).

However, as we have seen, NDE are not always the same from a cross-cultural point of view. For instance Allan Kellehear after having completed a number of extensive reviews of NDEs in both Western and non-Western countries (Kellehear 1993, 1996, 2008), suggested that only two features of the NDEs are present cross-culturally:

- the transition into a period of darkness

- the meeting with 'other beings', once arrived in the 'other world'.

Other aspects, like a 'life review', are nearly always absent in non-Western accounts. Others argued that the only common element among different cultures is the spatial element of 'being in a place' (Corazza 2010). According to this view, the intuition of their own death, reported by those who had an NDE, made them lose interest in time, which for them no longer existed, although time gradually regained meaning after recovery. By contrast, the spatial characteristic of 'being in a place' with specific qualities is always present throughout the experiences and acquired a deeper significance. Although the 'transcendent' places visited during the experiences varied from heavenly gardens to open sepulchers, from rural villages to forests, no single account was 'placeless' (Corazza 2008, 2010). Belanti, Perera and Jagadheesan (2008) examined cross-cultural aspects of NDE using a phenomenological approach. They commented on the rich interplay of many factors that come to bear, when an individual narrates her/his experience. They were of the opinion that, 'Although there may be a core component to NDE, cultural influences must be considered when attempting to interpret individual narratives' (p.130).

It is crucial to observe that the cultural comparison between NDEs in different countries is a very difficult topic of investigation, especially in the absence of extensive data as well as a deep understanding of the linguistic structure of the time period in which the NDE was described. However, we would like to suggest that there are certain cognitive structures (or 'eidetic essences') that are common to all cultures, independently from what has been experienced. These might include the sense of:

- realness: the conviction that what happened was a real experience and not an hallucination

- transcendence: the experience of visiting another world, or plane of consciousness

- transformation: the experience had some important life-changing effects in life-path, or personal beliefs, usually in a more spiritual sense

- value/originality: the experience was one of the more important experiences of their life.

Conclusion

From the accounts around the globe it is apparent that the NDE is a universal phenomenon encountered in various situations both clinical and otherwise. Cultural factors and the belief systems appear to be influencing the presentation. It appears that the phenomenon can occur in almost any religious background and there is usually a change in attitudes, belief systems and behaviour of individuals following similar experiences. Clinicians need to be aware that NDEs may occur in order to identify patients with such experiences. Patients with NDE may not initially divulge the story to the clinicians thinking that they may not believe this 'unusual experience' or due to the fear of being ridiculed or even stigmatized as 'mentally insane'. Awareness of this phenomenon amongst the clinicians and more importantly in our context an understanding of the cultural overtones, therefore, is necessary in order to elicit such information and help the NDEr who may be mystified by what has happened. There are clear differences in the experiences of individuals from different walks of life. There are common elements as well. It behoves the listener to give the individual a 'safe' environment in which he/she is enabled to ventilate their thoughts. A therapist would need to listen with empathy rather than in a perfunctory manner. This is important especially when it is a fearful NDE. With the ready availability of travel and the mass movement of people around the globe, one may be a stranger (due to the NDE) not only in their own country but in a far and distant land. Not listening with empathy could add insult to injury. Once more the understanding of the therapist will help assuage their anxiety. There needs to be a formulation of what was experienced in relation to their culture, religious beliefs, etc. and the individual needs to be helped to make sense of what has taken place. If a therapist is uncertain or lacks the knowledge required then help may be sought from an established person from that community to which the NDEr belongs. We need to bear in mind that even with people in their own country there are different religious beliefs, cultural practices and language itself. Accessing such a person may take place either face to face or by telephone, a video conference or other technological means.

CHAPTER 5

Near-Death Experiences of Children

CHERIE SUTHERLAND

From the time Raymond Moody first published *Life After Life* in 1975 people have been fascinated by the near-death experience (NDE). However, the NDEs of children rarely rated a mention until 1983 when Melvin Morse published the now well-known case of a seven-year-old near-drowning victim. Morse (Morse and Perry 1990) had resuscitated this child, whom he later called Katie, in the emergency room of a nearby hospital. Two weeks later during a follow-up appointment, when Morse attempted to identify the circumstances of Katie's near drowning by asking what she remembered from the experience, she replied, 'Do you mean when I visited the heavenly Father?' She then became embarrassed and would go no further with her story.

One week later, however, during another visit, Katie described travelling through a dark tunnel, which became bright when a tall woman 'with bright yellow hair' appeared. This other-worldly guide, Elizabeth, accompanied Katie into heaven, where she encountered deceased relatives and even two souls awaiting rebirth; and then she met 'the heavenly Father and Jesus'. After being asked if she wanted to see her mother again, she said 'yes' and woke up in her body. Despite being amazed by what he heard, Morse later wrote that she had told her story in such a 'powerful and compelling' way, he believed her implicitly (p.7).

Soon after the publication of Morse's article, Nancy Evans Bush (1983) reported 17 accounts of NDEs in children, and in 1984, Glen Gabbard and Stuart Twemlow – who, himself, had had an NDE as a child – published three more cases in *With the Eyes of the Mind*. Even in 1990, at the time Melvin Morse with Paul Perry published *Closer to the Light*, the number of child NDE accounts was still small (Herzog and Herrin 1985; Morse, Castillo, Venecia, Milstein, and Tyler 1986; Morse, Conner, and Tyler 1985; Serdahely 1987–88, 1989–90, 1990; Serdahely and Walker 1990a, b).

Because *Closer to the Light* was the first book devoted exclusively to the NDEs of children, and was readily available to the media and wider public alike, its contents were both enthusiastically welcomed and vigorously debated. There was also a growing interest in child NDErs among researchers such as Gabbard and Twemlow (1984) and Irwin (1989), because it was believed that the accounts of children, especially very young ones, would be relatively free of cultural influence. Other books with a focus on this population soon followed (Steiger and Steiger 1995; Sutherland 1995), further adding to the pool of child NDE accounts.

Comparison of adult and child experiences

There is no doubt that every NDE is unique. However, underpinning this unique expression are the deep structures of the typical NDE pattern. It is particularly interesting to see this pattern played out in the multiple experiences of people who have had NDEs both as children and adults. As they relate their stories, it becomes clear that the form or complexity of the experience has no discernible relationship to the age of the experiencer. One example is the case of Hannah, which I reported in *Children of the Light* (1995). Hannah had four NDEs: two in early childhood, one as a teenager, and another at age 20 during childbirth. Hannah related her story as follows:

> I was born a Jew in Germany probably some time in late 1937
> ... My first experience happened when I was 3 or 4 years
> old. I remember being taken out of my house by my father
> and a soldier ... I looked back and saw my mother yelling

... an SS officer went over to her ... and shot her in the head with his pistol ... I screamed. He turned, raised the pistol and pointed it at me. I turned to run and was shot in the back. I experienced a shock ... Then I heard music. I can't describe it in earthly terms. I was in darkness, then the darkness changed into a passage and then it was light and peaceful, like being in a big smile. I heard voices and ... in the light I saw 'beings' ... I tried to reach out to one. Tears were in his eyes ... At that moment the pain started, and I must have slipped into a state of sleep or unconsciousness (Sutherland 1995, pp.142–143)

Upon regaining consciousness some time later, Hannah realized she had been taken to the nuns, who were looking after her. Doctors began to operate on her back. She said:

I faded out. It was blue-black then a roaring black, then once again there was peace. This time there was no music, no lullaby. I saw two people I knew but I don't remember their relationship, and I also saw three 'beings'. The third 'being' then sent me a message of hope, love, and caring. He sent me messages of a future without pain. (p.144)

She assumes she then returned to her body, because later, while strapped in splints, she remembers the building being on fire and being rescued by being thrown out the window. Before the end of the war Hannah was taken to New Zealand as an orphan, and her next NDE occurred when she was about 15 in a bicycle accident. This time she had no awareness of any darkness or pain, but while out-of-body she observed the people who were gathered around her. She said, 'I floated happily, watching myself and them for a very long time' (p.144).

Five years later, at 20, while afflicted with pneumonia and heavily pregnant, she was rushed to the hospital. Her child was born in a great hurry. She said, 'I could see her, myself, and the doctors and nurses, and then I travelled through the tunnel until I was presented with the choice of rest or going back' (p.145). The next thing she knew, she was in the Intensive Care Unit, and three days later her daughter died.

Reliability of retrospective accounts

The earliest of Hannah's NDEs was recounted to me 50 years after the event. This time lapse raises two fundamental questions:

- How reliable are such retrospective accounts?

- How affected by cultural conditioning and social expectations are their contents?

In Western societies, in our present secular age, the level of religious training received by young people is often rudimentary at best. It is for this reason that researchers have taken an interest in the NDEs of young children. However, many investigators have disputed the 'cultural conditioning' argument (e.g. Bush 1983; Gabbard and Twemlow 1984; Morse 1983; Serdahely 1991). And I have come across several cases myself in which the children specifically commented on how *different* certain aspects of their experiences were from what they were led to expect from their religious or cultural background. As Richard Bonenfant (2001) pointed out, 'Children's accounts are often informative simply because they report exactly what they see without great concern over the rational interpretation of their observations' (p.95). Their accounts seem untainted. However, implicit in this thinking is the questionable notion that the accounts of adults are substantially different from those of children and are overly determined by religion and culture.

In the case of Hannah, who reported both childhood and adult NDEs, there is no evidence that she embellished her childhood experiences over time to conform with adult notions of rationality or cultural acceptability. Indeed I found that adults often described their childhood NDEs in child-like terms. One of my interviewees, Barbara, described the amazement she felt while out-of-body:

> I was floating on the ceiling and I was just so, so happy … and my first thought was, 'How mean of them not to tell me about this before!' … And then I began to look around. There were two old-fashioned wardrobes in the room, and I thought, 'Oh gee, Mother doesn't dust the top very well. I can write my name in this.' I was enjoying just bouncing around … But then I thought, 'Now I'm going!' (Sutherland 1993, p.25)

Barbara told me the feeling she had was better than 'all the birthday parties' she'd ever been to. This is not a child speaking but rather a 62-year-old woman who, as a ten-year-old child, had been critically ill with pneumonia. Her child-like curiosity and thoughts, the emotion in her voice, and the tears in her eyes as she related her story, convinced me absolutely that she was presenting the account exactly as she had experienced it so many years before.

William Serdahely, in his comparison of retrospective and contemporary accounts of childhood NDEs (1991), concluded that adult retrospective accounts were indistinguishable from contemporary pediatric NDEs (p.223). This finding supported earlier work by Bush (1983). And in discussing his own results, Morse wrote, 'Unlike ordinary memories or dreams, NDEs do not seem to be rearranged or altered over time' (Morse 1994b, p.142).

The NDEs of very young children

It has often been supposed that the NDEs of very young children will have a content limited to their vocabulary. However, it is now clear that the age of children at the time of their NDE does not in any way determine its complexity. Even pre-linguistic children have later reported quite complex experiences. For instance, Marcella, who was ten years old when I interviewed her, described the NDE she had on the first day of life when born prematurely, one of twins, and dangerously tiny. She said:

> I remember ... I saw a light ... and there was this head in the light. And behind me there was this other man who was trying to get me to go back to reality. But he [the head in the light] was trying to make me stay. Then I saw this girl walking into the light and this man told me, 'Why don't you be like her ... When you get to the end you'll find a surprise." So I decided I'd walk behind her.
>
> In the background of the head ... were all these little bubbles full of light and every time he moved one of them burst ... and all this gold and coloured air came out. I was frightened at first but then ... I wasn't scared any more. I would have liked to stay.
>
> But before I got right into the light ... there was some type of force that was taking me back. I could see the colours coming towards me ... and then that's all I remember, I just went back into my body. (Sutherland 1995, pp.82–83)

In *Lessons from the Light* (2000) Kenneth Ring and Evelyn Elsaesser Valarino explored research on perinatal memory reported by David B. Chamberlain, a psychologist and perinatal researcher. As a result of his extensive inquiry, he became convinced absolutely that birth memories are often genuine recollections of actual experiences. According to Chamberlain, objections based on assumptions that the brains of newborns are insufficiently developed to process such memories are unfounded (Ring and Valarino 2000, pp.116–117).

Ring and Valarino (2000) related the story of Mark Botts, who, aged nine months, suffering from severe bronchiolitis, had his NDE during a full cardiopulmonary arrest. It apparently took more than 40 minutes for doctors to revive him, and afterwards he was in a coma for an additional three months. One day, more than four years later, totally without warning or previous reference, he surprised his parents by talking about 'when he had died'. He described how, during his experience, he left his body and crawled through a dark tunnel into a bright golden light where he was greeted warmly by some 'white clouded figures'. He then glided down a golden road until suddenly a being whom he understood to be God, appeared in front of him. They conversed telepathically until Mark was sent back (pp.108–112).

Such stories, according to Peter Fenwick and Elizabeth Fenwick (1995), are significant because they clearly indicate that 'the NDE does not depend on the maturation and development of the brain' and possibly even that NDEs 'reflect some fundamental features of experience to which the dying brain, *at any age*, has access' (pp.182–183).

The circumstances

Just as age does not seem in any way to affect the content of the NDE, neither does the nature of the near-death crisis appear to be a significant determinant of NDEs in general. Some hospital-based studies have been focused on a particular precipitating factor, such as cardiac arrest (Greyson 2003; Holden and Joesten 1990; Parnia *et al.* 2001; Sabom 1982; Schwaninger *et al.* 2002; van Lommel *et al.* 2001) or meningococcal disease (Shears *et al.* 2002), but most research has drawn on people who have had their NDEs in a diverse range of circumstances: illness, surgery, accidents and drowning, suicide (Colli and Beck 2003; Rosen 1975; Sutherland 1993), and violence such as war traumas (Sutherland 1995), sexual abuse (Serdahely 1987–88, 1992, 1993), and physical abuse of various kinds (Sutherland 1995).

In *The Omega Project*, Ring (1992) asserted that NDErs are more likely than others to have had a history of child abuse and other childhood traumas (p.143). This claim has been widely discussed (Hoffman 1998; Morse and Perry 1992; Morse 1994a; Serdahely 1992, 1993). In an earlier article, Ring and Christopher Rosing (1990) postulated that such a background of abuse or trauma would tend to foster a defensive 'dissociative response style', and in near-death crisis situations promote sensitivity to NDEs (p.231). They write, 'such persons are what we might call psychological sensitives with low stress thresholds, and it is their traumatic childhoods that have helped to make them that way' (p. 232).

The content of NDEs in children and teens

Affect

The most commonly reported feature of NDEs is a sense of peace and well-being – all-encompassing love and tranquillity. However, there can also be moments of excitement, elation, fun, curiosity, puzzlement, and even fear.

Leaving the body

Typically, as a feature of the NDE, the out-of-body experience is often the NDEr's first indication that something is wrong. Tommy, who was eight years old when he suffered a ruptured spleen and closed head injury during a car accident was on life support for 21 days and then in a coma for three months. Five and a half years after his near-death crisis, he still suffered considerable physical disabilities, his speech was still affected, and his mental development had been retarded. Nonetheless, he was keen to describe to me his experience of being out-of-body. He said, 'I felt like ... my inner body was taken out of me ... I felt like a dummy almost, that my body was like a dummy and I was outside it' (Sutherland 1995, p.68).

Elisabeth Kübler-Ross (1983) maintained that 'children who are in a coma are out of their physical body most of the time, and during this time they can hear all communications that people may have with them' (p.59). During the months he was comatose, Tommy's parents communicated with him constantly – hopeful he *would* hear them and be comforted – yet they were not prepared for just how much he had *observed* while out of his body.

Moving through the darkness towards the light

Once out of the body, typically the experiencer will travel through an area of darkness – usually described as a tunnel – towards a light. Even a pre-verbal or non-verbal child may give some indication that they have travelled through a tunnel. Herzog and Herrin (1985) recounted the story of an infant of six months who had been admitted to the Intensive Care Unit (ICU). They noted that some months later 'she had a panic reaction when encouraged by her siblings to crawl through a tunnel at a local store' (p.1074). Apparently this 'tunnel panic' reaction had occurred on other occasions, too. Then, three years after the child's hospitalization, when her mother was explaining the imminent death of the grandmother, the child asked, 'Will Grandma have to go through the tunnel at the store to get to see God?'(p.1074).

One of the distinctive features of children's NDEs is that they are often accompanied by a luminous presence as they travel through the tunnel into the light. Although this loving being is often called an 'angel' it can also be described as a 'beautiful lady' or 'light figure' of some kind.

Life review

The angelic being may also be in attendance as the child experiences a life review, providing loving support and encouragement when needed. Some children receive a message about the future – a phenomenon Ring (1985) called a 'personal flashforward' (p.183) – and it often occurs while the experiencers are deciding whether or not to stay in the other world. For instance, Natalie, 15 years old, was shown how sad her mother would be if she died (Serdahely 1990, p.35) and this influenced her decision to return.

Another common flashforward is for the child to be given a 'mission'. For instance, Dorothea, 51 years old, was only five when she nearly drowned. During her NDE a voice said to her, 'I have work for you' (Sutherland 1995, p.29). Dorothea told me that she had never forgotten this message and had always had it at the forefront of her mind when making choices at various times throughout her life. These choices had led her to train as a nurse, and when I first met her she had already been working for some years with aboriginal people in a desert community.

Encountering others

As in Dorothea's case, the encounter can sometimes be auditory rather than visual; however, in the NDEs of many children, the voice is also embodied, particularly once they reach the 'world of light'. The spiritual beings most frequently reported by children are angels or light beings, as we have already seen, deceased relatives or friends, Jesus, and The Light or God.

Coming back

All these children at some point returned. Some chose to come back, others were sent back, and some just suddenly found themselves back in their bodies. For those who remember being sent back, the feeling of rejection can, at first, be overwhelming. Children and teens in such circumstances often wonder what is wrong with them. Why are they being sent away? Why are they being punished? To be abruptly torn away from an experience of bliss and returned to a painful body can be overwhelming. And if their attempts to talk about their experiences are dismissed, the repercussions can be long lasting.

Telling others

Many children try to tell someone about their experience quite soon after the event, and the response they receive appears to greatly influence how they subsequently think about it. If they are believed, this acknowledgement can help begin the integration process and provide an impetus for ongoing change and personal growth (Sutherland 1992). Unfortunately, not everyone is so blessed. Many children, when rebuffed, end up keeping silent. For instance, Hal, who was 14 years old when he had several cardiac arrests, said,

> I tried to tell my mother and was told, 'Don't be silly'. I tried
> to tell my scoutmaster and my local Methodist minister. They
> seemed to be embarrassed. So I just stopped ... I just didn't
> tell anyone about it after that. (Sutherland 1995, p.186)

Carol Jean Morres, who was 14 years old when she had her NDE said, 'Because others cannot accept my experience as real, I have had to keep it locked up inside me for the most part, and that creates a feeling of isolation and loneliness' (Atwater 2003, p.95). Atwater (2003) stated that children are six times more likely than adults to 'tuck away' their experience (p.111). Although it is unclear how Atwater came to this conclusion, there are indeed many cases in the literature of children either totally forgetting their NDEs or putting them on hold until something triggers their memory or suddenly helps them come to an understanding of it (see Gabbard and Twemlow 1984, p.157; Sutherland 1993, p.89; 1995, p.186). However, even if children have never told anybody about their NDEs, the many after-effects that reverberate through their lives may well reveal their status as NDErs.

The aftermath

Probably the most universally experienced after-effect among any population of NDErs is the decline in death anxiety following their NDE (see Ring 1982; Sabom 1982). In my own study of 50 NDErs ranging in age from 7 to 76 years at the time of their experience, 98 per cent reported no fear of death following their NDE (1992, p.87). Morse and Perry (1992) wrote that this change is 'simply because they have been there and know what to expect' (p.64).

In a study comparing the after-effects reported by NDErs and non-NDErs, Bonenfant (2004) found that the majority of NDErs spoke of multiple after-effects that were ongoing and, in some cases, even increased over time. He even found statistically significant differences on spiritual and paranormal measures.

In my own study of after-effects, 76 per cent of my sample of 50 NDErs claimed to be spiritually inclined rather than religious after their NDEs (Sutherland 1992, p.99). Paranormal after-effects are also very common (see Ring 1985; Sutherland 1992). These phenomena can range from the enjoyable and playful to the quite disturbing. Some children have ongoing contact with deceased relatives (Sutherland 1995, p.41), and some speak of 'guardian angel' type figures that communicate with them (Atwater 2003, p.34; Liester 1998; Morse and Perry 1992, p.11). Some children are aware of things before they happen. This precognition can range from the easy-to-live-with knowing who is on the phone when it rings, to having dreams or visions that can be so distressing that the experiencer may want to have their ability removed (Fenwick and Fenwick 1995, p.147; Steiger and Steiger 1995, p.76). Some children have out-of-body experiences (Sutherland 1995, p.23), and some report knowing things about other people and reading minds (Sutherland 1995, p.41).

Child and teen NDErs also describe a number of other strange phenomena. For instance, some find they can never wear watches because they always break (Morse and Perry 1992, p.11). There can be an unusual sensitivity to light and sound and a generalized sensitivity to anything electrical (Atwater 2003, p.83). Bonenfant (2004) reported many examples of synesthesia such as 'feeling colors, tasting words or smelling sounds' (p.163). He found the incidence of such sensory confusion to be surprisingly high – two-thirds – among a population of NDErs ranging in age from 10 to 76 (p.171).

Yet, however surprising or confusing many of these specific after-effects may be for child experiencers, they still appear to be just additional symptoms reinforcing their overall feeling of being different when they come back – different from how they were before *and* different from everybody else. Many children describe feeling estranged from their peer group because they no longer share the same interests (Greyson 1997; Sutherland 1995, p.40). They tend to be indifferent to materialistic and competitive success and status (Flynn 1986). They've often had an experience of being 'all-knowing' or 'at-one-with-everything' and return with an overwhelming thirst for knowledge and meaning that can set them apart. Emily, ten years old, who had her NDE when she was five, actually said to her mother that she wished she could 'spend a day in some other child's body just to know what it felt like to be normal' (Sutherland 1995, p.79).

For some families, dealing with a child NDEr can be very challenging. My first contact with Emily's mother occurred when she wrote to me seeking advice on how to handle the turmoil in her family caused by Emily's NDE and its aftermath. She wrote that when Emily told her about her experience, she was shocked. She continued:

> She was very different from the small child I knew before the illness but I had no idea why ... Last year Emily had a very bad time ... Up until that point she had been a loner but that awful year led her to depend more on her peers, and it upset her to discover just how different she was from other children. (Sutherland 1995, p.74)

Emily's mother then related how she had begun reading to her from one of my books, and had discussed 'many key bits' with her. As a result, she wrote, 'Acceptance has begun to replace her confusion, self-doubt, low self-esteem and feelings of mental instability as she now knows she is not alone' (Sutherland 1995, p.75).

The experience of Emily's mother strongly suggests that parents – and perhaps others such as health care professionals, or indeed anyone who is knowledgeable about NDEs and their after-effects – can critically influence the relative amount of distress or peace of mind, or even developmental enhancement a child will experience in the aftermath of an NDE.

Help for the dying and grieving

Beliefs and knowledge can also have a major influence on the nature and duration of the grieving process (see Sutherland 1997). Many bereaved parents contacted me after the publication of my first book to tell me of the solace they had found in the NDEs of children following the death of their child. Marja, whose five-year-old son had died in a drowning accident, told me that when she serendipitously came across an account of a childhood near-drowning NDE in a German magazine, she felt totally exhilarated. From that day on, she read everything she could find about NDEs, and, she said, 'with each new account, the bottomless, black despair I had felt for so long receded' (Sutherland 1995, p.6).

Bruce Horacek (1997), describing the NDE as a 'healing gift', outlined several situations in which having an NDE, or knowledge of NDEs and other death-related visions, can be helpful in facing one's own death or the death of a significant other. Indeed, many childhood NDErs have told me that as adults they have gone on to work with the dying or grieving. Having no fear of death themselves appears to give NDErs the confidence to ease that fear in others.

Knowledge of NDEs even has the potential to help health care professionals who work with terminally ill children. As Morse (1994a) suggested, rather than viewing death as a professional defeat and doing everything possible to prevent it from happening, if NDEs and other death-related visions were to be taken into account, the heroic measures often put in place – utilizing expensive, intrusive, dehumanizing medical procedures on dying patients without any real hope of prolonging life – could be drastically reduced (p.82).

Helping child NDErs

It is important to be aware that any patient, even a young child, might have had an NDE during a health crisis situation. During any period of unconsciousness it should be assumed that paediatric patients can still see and hear, and even feel what is going on around their body. During the crisis, Manley (1996) suggests that one member of the team should be stationed at the patient's head to provide an ongoing commentary, and simple explanation of procedures. She also recommends encouraging the family to be present – both during and following a critical event. During a crisis, the touch of a parent can 'ground' the child and encourage them to return, while afterwards, frequent touching can help to reorient them to their body (Manley 1996, p.316). Once regaining consciousness the child can be feeling vulnerable and disoriented, so it is vital not to abandon them at that point (Corcoran 1988, p.39).

When children tell nurses or other health care professionals about NDEs the timing is typically either during or immediately following resuscitation, that is, the closer someone has been to death the more likely they are to make such a report. As Morse writes:

> The scientific evidence clearly suggests that NDEs occur when they are subjectively perceived as occurring, at the point of death. As such, they must represent the best objective evidence of what it is like to die, regardless of which neurotransmitters or anatomical structures mediate the experience. (1994b, p.143)

It is therefore important for health care professionals such as emergency department staff, and for that matter, anyone working with dying patients, to thoroughly inform themselves, and be willing to explore their own attitudes to NDEs and other paranormal phenomena associated with the dying process (Corcoran 1988, p.38).

They need to be alert for any signs that a patient may have had an NDE (Corcoran 1988, p.38; Manley 1996, p.316). These could range from withdrawal (the need to be quiet and reflect on what has happened), to elation, excitement, and even sadness or anger (in cases where they have been sent back against their will, or jolted prematurely from their experience by successful resuscitation). It is possible the child will say something like 'I've just had the strangest dream', or 'I've just been to heaven', and then wait for a response. If the nurse or doctor says, 'Oh, don't be silly, you're all right now!' or makes some other such response, it is highly unlikely that an NDEr will proceed with an account of the experience. However, if they are met with interest, and acceptance of the reality of the experience, it is much more likely that an NDE will be disclosed (Sutherland 1991, p.13).

Whatever their personal beliefs, health care professionals need to be willing to listen attentively and without judgement to any reports, however vaguely they may be expressed. They need to respect the perspective and interpretation of the child NDEr (Corcoran 1988, p.38; Manley 1996, p.316) however young they might be. As Susan Schoenbeck cautions, 'Don't assume your patient is confused . . . Try to assume a reflective rather than an analytical stance' (1993, p.46). It is important just to listen, not analyse, or attempt to 'explain away' the experience, however distressed the experiencer may appear to be. Near-death experiencers need to be able to freely express whatever emotions they might be feeling (Corcoran 1988, p.38). Such an event can be a huge shock, quite apart from the affront to their physical body.

And as their physical condition improves, if given the opportunity, child NDErs often like to draw their experience (Manley 1996, p.316). While interviewing children, and even young teens, I always found that as soon as they had coloured pens and paper in front of them they began to relax and share their experiences without reservation, often giving a running commentary as they giggled about their lack of artistic talent, or focused fixedly on their drawings. Even those who had been all but inarticulate before the pens and paper appeared could be quite forthcoming.

If asked, it is important to provide accurate information about NDEs to both the child and their parents. Most like to read of other people's experiences but it is equally important not to force it on them if they don't appear interested. Morse comments that parents and family also need to be 'reassured that such experiences are common, normal, and not the result of medications, high fevers, or brain pathology' (1994b p.143).

It can be helpful to counsel parents on the likely after-effects since even if these are positive, the family can still be stressed by the child's change in personality and priorities (Manley 1996, p.316). In most cases, it is not necessary to refer the child for further counselling, although for children and teens disturbed by their experience, indeed in any case of emotional fragility, it can be helpful for them to speak with a counsellor experienced in working with NDErs, or at the very least, familiar with the literature (Bonenfant 2001; Bush 2002; Greyson 1997).

The NDE is a profound, emotionally powerful experience. As illustrated in the case of Emily's mother, perhaps the best way to be of service to a child experiencer is simply to be informed, aware, sensitive, interested, and willing to give support. However, the importance of validating the experience cannot be overemphasized, because this sort of acknowledgement is an important first step on the child's integration trajectory (Sutherland 1992). Nowhere has this principle been more clearly demonstrated than in the case of David, a non-verbal quadriplegic adolescent who was assisted over a period of many months by social worker Rick Enright (2004) in the arduous task of revealing his NDE. Enright concluded that, for David, this revelation – and having it acknowledged – was an incredibly important process, which 'brought about significant changes in his emotional state, helped return personal control over his life, and ultimately led to his peaceful and fulfilling death' (p.195).

Conclusion

After more than 30 years of research we now know that children of all ages are capable of having, *and remembering*, NDEs. And there can no longer be any doubt that these peak experiences 'leave profound and transformative effects in their wake' (Hoffman 1998, p.2).

In terms of NDE content, even though every experience is unique, the NDEs of children and teens follow a consistent pattern that appears to be little different from the pattern experienced by adults – *including* the presence of a life review. And neither do children's experiences appear to be affected by cause of near-death crisis, age, gender, religiosity, or any other demographic variable. One distinction appears to be that children are almost always accompanied into the light. Although adults do also sometimes have the sense of a presence with them early in their experience, children seem far more often to see, and even to have their hand held by, a luminous being of one kind or another as they move together into the other world. We know that children – even very young children – can have distressing moments in their experiences, yet overall, as in adults, the experience is primarily a pleasurable one.

In terms of after-effects, the range is so wide and varied – including physiological, neurophysiological, psychological, emotional, social, behavioural, attitudinal, spiritual, and paranormal – that it is impossible to make a blanket statement about them, other than to say that people around child and teen experiencers frequently comment on how changed those children are after their NDEs. And overall, despite an initial period of turmoil and problems of adjustment, over time, many of the after-effects *are* successfully integrated and experienced as positive.

In summary, clinicians need to be aware that NDEs do occur in childhood and if they want to assist them in dealing with the experience and its consequences they must be willing to approach children with patience and empathy, taking into account the possible limitations of their linguistic ability and their sometimes idiosyncratic ways of telling their stories.

Although it has now been shown that childhood NDEs related by adults many years later are reliable – not distorted or altered to fit in with cultural or social expectations – to hear those same stories from a child is a special privilege. One can learn again and again from their accounts that there is no need to fear death because death is not an ending but rather a transition into another realm. Daniel, aged 14 years, who was born with severe birth defects and had 17 major operations and many NDEs in his early years, said, 'Death's all right. I know I could die any time so I just live each day. I'd say to people who are dying, "Don't be afraid. It's a beautiful place"' (Sutherland 1995, p.105).

CHAPTER 6

Pathophysiological Aspects of Near-Death Experiences

PIM VAN LOMMEL

To study the abnormal is the best way of understanding the normal. (William James 1958)

Introduction

As a cardiologist I have had the privilege to meet many patients who were willing to share their near-death experience (NDE) with me. The first time this happened was in 1969. In the coronary care unit the alarm suddenly went off. A patient was going into cardiac arrest. After two electric shocks and a spell of unconsciousness lasting some four minutes, the patient regained consciousness, much to the relief of the nursing staff and attendant doctor. I had just started my cardiology training that year, and that attendant doctor was me. Following the successful resuscitation everyone was pleased, except the patient. To everyone's surprise the patient was extremely disappointed. He spoke of a tunnel, of colours, of a light, of a beautiful landscape and of music. He was extremely emotional. The term 'near-death experience' did not yet exist, nor had I ever heard of people having any recollection of the period of their cardiac arrest. Whilst studying for my degree, I had learnt that such a thing is in fact impossible: being unconscious means not being aware, and that applies to people suffering a cardiac arrest or patients in a coma. The fact that people report lucid experiences in their consciousness during cardiac arrest or coma is difficult to reconcile with current medical opinion. An NDE is a special state of enhanced consciousness that occurs during an imminent or actual period of death, or sometimes without any obvious reason. The paradoxical occurrence of heightened, lucid awareness and logical thought processes during a period of impaired cerebral perfusion raises particular perplexing questions for our current understanding of consciousness and its relation to brain function. A clear sensorium and complex perceptual processes during a period of apparent clinical death challenge the concept that consciousness is localized exclusively in the brain. When the brain is so dysfunctional that the patient is deeply comatose, those cerebral structures, which underpin subjective experience and memory, must be severely impaired, and complex experiences such as are reported in the NDE should not arise or be retained in memory. Such patients would be expected to have no subjective experience at all. Even hallucinations should not be possible in such circumstances.

According to mainstream science, it is quite impossible to find a scientific explanation for the NDE as long as we 'believe' that consciousness is only a side-effect of a functioning brain.

Theories regarding cause and content

Until recently there was no prospective and scientifically designed study to explain the cause and content of an NDE; all studies had been retrospective and very selective with respect to patients. Based on these incomplete retrospective studies some believed the experience could be caused by physiological changes in the brain as a result of lack of oxygen (cerebral anoxia); other theories encompass a psychological reaction to approaching death, hallucinations, dreams, side-effect of drugs, or just false memories. NDE are indeed reported under extremely diverse circumstances: not only in life-threatening situations, most frequently after severe impairment of brain function, but also in situations without any physical or psychological danger (see Table 6.1). And is there a reason why only a small number of patients, whether or not in a critical condition, report an NDE?

Table 6.1: Circumstances that may prompt an NDE (van Lommel 2010)

A. Brain function (seriously) impaired	B. Brain function unimpaired
Cardiac arrest in patients suffering a myocardial infarction or serious arrhythmia	Serious, but not immediately life-threatening, illnesses with high fever
Coma caused by brain damage after a traffic accident or brain haemorrhage	Isolation (e.g. shipwrecked people), extreme dehydration, or hypothermia
Coma caused by near-drowning, especially in children	Depression or existential crisis
Coma caused by diabetes, asphyxia, or apnea	Meditation
Coma caused by a failed suicide bid or intoxication	Without a clear medical indication, such as a walk in nature
Unconsciousness caused by shock (low blood pressure) as a result of	Similar experiences, so-called 'fear-death experiences', are reported after a seemingly inevitable death, such as an imminent traffic accident or a mountaineering accident.
• severe blood loss during or after a delivery, or during surgery	
• an allergic reaction	
• a serious infection (sepsis)	
Under general anaesthesia, usually following complications from surgery	
Electrocution (electric shock)	

Some NDE elements, specifically the lucid consciousness and verifiable perception during the loss or serious impairment of brain function, challenge the prevailing view of the relationship between consciousness and the brain, which sees consciousness as a product of brain function. This is why many scientists struggle to understand NDEs and why research into the subject can be seen as a threat to scientific dogma. This is perhaps why still many scientists assume that an NDE is caused by oxygen deficiency in the brain. Many scientists would attempt to explain the NDE with the help of existing theories and models and often end up giving perhaps a rather one-sided and simplified account of the NDE in an attempt to reconcile the comprehensive phenomenon with existing approaches. This has resulted in theories that can account for one or more aspects of the NDE, but not for the complex phenomenon in its entirety. However, it is highly likely that the brain plays some role in all of this, because certain NDE-like phenomena can be induced by stimulating a particular place in the brains of epileptics. This is why I will summarize the most commonly mentioned physiological views about the cause and content of an NDE.

Physiological theories
OXYGEN DEFICIENCY
When a cardiac arrest disrupts the blood flow to the brain, the result is unconsciousness due to the total cessation of oxygen supply to the brain (anoxia). Breathing stops, all physical and brainstem reflexes cease, and unless resuscitation is initiated within five to ten minutes patients will die. However, in the case of oxygen *deficiency* in the brain (hypoxia), as seen in low blood pressure (shock), heart failure or asphyxia, the result is not unconsciousness but confusion and agitation. Brain damage after waking from a coma is also associated with confusion, fear, agitation, memory defects, and muddled speech.

A study of fighter jet pilots is often cited as a possible explanatory model for NDE. Having been placed in a centrifuge, these pilots experienced momentary oxygen deficiency in the brain when the enormous increase in gravity caused their blood to drop to their feet. Fighter jet pilots can indeed lose consciousness, and often experience convulsions, like those seen in epilepsy, or tingling around the mouth and in the arms and legs, as well as confusion upon waking. Sometimes they also experience some elements that are reminiscent of an NDE, such as a kind of tunnel vision, a sensation of light, a peaceful sense of floating, or the observation of brief, fragmented images from the past (Whinnery and Whinnery 1990). They seldom also see images of living persons, but never of deceased people. There are no reports of a life review or out-of-body episodes.

A similar kind of unconsciousness, sometimes accompanied by the experiences reported by pilots, occurs after fainting induced by hyperventilation, followed by a so-called Valsalva manoeuvre (Lempert, Bauer and Schmidt 1994). The latter involves trying to push air from the body with the mouth and nose closed, which slows the heartbeat and lowers blood pressure, and results in a short-lived oxygen deficiency in the brain. The effects of this type of faint have also been wrongly compared to an NDE (Lempert *et al.* 1994). Nonetheless, the most common explanation for NDE is an extremely severe and life-threatening oxygen deficiency in the brain, resulting in a brief spell of abnormal brain activity, followed by reduced activity and, finally, the loss of all brain activity. This theory seems inapplicable however, because an NDE is actually accompanied by an enhanced and lucid consciousness with memories, and because it can also be experienced under circumstances such as an imminent traffic accident or a depression, neither of which involves oxygen deficiency. Moreover, in an out-of-body experience (OBE) patients have *during* the period of their resuscitation perceptions from a position outside and above their lifeless body, and doctors, nurses, and relatives can later verify the reported perceptions, and they can also corroborate the precise moment the NDE with out-of-body experience occurred *during* the period of cardiopulmonary resuscitation (CPR).

CARBON-DIOXIDE OVERLOAD

Oxygen deficiency is accompanied by an increase in carbon-dioxide (CO_2) in the body. This increased level of carbon-dioxide in the blood has been cited as a possible cause of NDE. Over 50 years ago, Meduna (1950) asked people to breathe in CO_2. Some experienced a sense of separation from the body, with occasional reports of a bright light, a tunnel, a sense of peace, or memory flashes. These images were quite rare, usually extremely fragmented, and never involved a life review or an encounter with deceased persons. Nor was it followed by a process of change. In other words, the inhalation of carbon-dioxide does not cause some of the characteristic NDE elements. One practical problem is that during a frantic resuscitation it is difficult to measure these gases (oxygen and carbon-dioxide) in the blood and impossible to measure them in the blood vessels in the brain. On the rare occasion when blood gases have been measured during resuscitation, it was usually only once the heartbeat and blood pressure had been stabilized, with the patient still unconscious on a ventilator and receiving extra oxygen.

In these cases the blood sample was taken from a vein or an artery in the arm or leg, and if the patient had an NDE, the level of oxygen saturation in the blood had been exceptionally high and the level of carbon-dioxide extremely low.

Klemenc-Ketis, Kersnik and Gremec (2010) published a study regarding 52 survivors of cardiac arrest, where 21 per cent reported an NDE, and where a significant correlation was found between higher initial partial pressures of end-tidal (Pet) CO_2, the level of Co_2 released at the end of expiration, and with higher arterial blood pressures of CO_2. However, this study included only patients with an out-of-hospital cardiac arrest, where arterial blood samples were taken only in the first five minutes after admission, meaning that most of them already had rhythm and blood pressure after successful CPR outside the hospital. It was not mentioned how accurate and when the end-tidal CO_2 was measured during and after the cardiac arrest and during the transport to the hospital. Besides, if they had corrected their statistics for multiple simultaneous univariate tests, none of the differences would have been significant because of the small sample size. Their main conclusion was that high levels of CO_2 in the blood in this study were associated with a very slightly higher incidence of NDEs, and this does not explain why the majority of patients with high CO_2 still not report an NDE. Moreover, Pet CO_2 has been shown to be a reliable and non-invasive prognostic indicator for a successful cardiac resuscitation, and highly correlates with cardiac index (Kolar *et al.* 2008; Saunders *et al.* 1989). So, the conclusion that high CO_2 levels could explain the causation of an NDE seems to be a questionable preliminary hypothesis.

Chemical reactions in the brain

KETAMINE

Because low doses of ketamine, a drug formerly used as an anaesthetic, can cause hallucinations, it has been postulated that this kind of substance is released in the brain during a period of stress or oxygen deficiency. Ketamine produces hallucinations because it blocks NMDA-receptors in the brain. A small quantity of ketamine gives some people a sense of detachment from the body or tunnel experiences (Jansen 1996). There are no known reports of an encounter with deceased persons or of a life review, nor have there been reports of positive changes. Ketamine usually causes such frightful and bizarre images, which are recognized as hallucinations, that research subjects prefer not to have the substance administered a second time. Because naturally occurring ketamine-like substances have never been found in the brain, this potential explanation must be abandoned. However, we cannot rule out that in some cases the blockade or malfunction of NMDA-receptors may play a role in the experience of an NDE.

ENDORPHIN

One of the first attempts at explaining an NDE was based on the fact that stress releases endorphin. This type of endogenous morphine occurs naturally in the body in small quantities and functions as a neurotransmitter. The substance is released in large quantities during stress. Endorphin can indeed get rid of pain and cause a sense of peace and well-being. However, the effects of endorphin usually last several hours, whereas the absence of pain and the sense of peace during an NDE vanish immediately after regaining consciousness. Endorphin also fails to explain other elements of an NDE.

PSYCHEDELICS (DIMETHYL TRIPTAMINE (DMT), LYSERGIC ACID DIETHYLAMIDE (LSD), PSILOCYBIN, AND MESCALINE)

These psychoactive substances are closely related to the neurotransmitter serotonin, which is found in large amounts in the body, and their chemical structure derives from tryptamine. These psychedelic substances have the same S2 receptor binding site in the brain as serotonin. DMT is produced in the pineal gland. This epiphysis, which does not consist of brain tissue, is close to the emotional, visual, and auditory centers of the brain and transmits its substances directly to both the brain and the blood. The substances produced in this gland are responsible for regulating the body's water balance and sleep–wake rhythm, and for developing the sexual glands until puberty. Perhaps they also play a role in dreams. The epiphysis also contains substances that can convert serotonin into DMT, and substances capable of blocking the enzymatic breakdown of DMT. The latter also occur in plants, and because it greatly enhances the effect of DMT the combination is used in ayahuasca (an Amazonian indigenous brew, traditionally used for shamanic, spiritual and healing purposes) in the Amazon (Strassman 2001).

The experience induced by psychoactive substances is sometimes similar to an NDE, especially in the case of DMT, although, depending on the dosage, confusing or frightening perceptions may also occur. These substance-induced experiences include the following elements: a sense of detachment from the body, out-of-body experiences, lucid and accelerated thought, an encounter with a being of light, a sense of unconditional love, being in an unearthly environment, access to a profound wisdom, and wordless communication with 'immaterial' beings. Sometimes the characteristic post-NDE transformation, including the loss of the fear of death, is also reported after administration of DMT (Strassman 2001) or LSD (Grof and Halifax 1977).

Electrical activity of the brain

EPILEPSY

An epileptic seizure is characterized by a kind of electrical storm, a short-circuit, which wipes out the electrical (and magnetic) activity in a certain area of the brain. As a result, normal activity of the brain cells (neurons) is blocked in that part of the cerebral cortex where the epileptic seizure originated. An epileptic seizure that originates in an area of the brain close to the temporal bone, the temporal lobes, may trigger muddled observations, mystical feelings, *déjà vu* experiences, a sense of detachment from the body (never an out-of-body experience with veridical perception), and olfactory or visual hallucinations. Sometimes these seizures are accompanied by unconsciousness or involuntary movements. After such an epileptic seizure of the temporal lobe, most patients have no memory of what happened to their bodies. They only remember what happened in their minds.

On the basis of these data some researchers have proposed a link between the NDE and either an increased activity or the cessation of all activity in the brain's temporal lobes. But studies with both superficial and deeper electrodes have shown that the symptoms of temporal lobe epilepsy are 'caused' by underlying (limbic) structures and not by the cerebral cortex itself. A detailed study among epileptic patients has also shown that the characteristic elements of an NDE are rarely mentioned after an epileptic seizure of the temporal lobe (Rodin 1989). Some elements are quite similar to an NDE, but *déjà vu* experiences are also frequently mentioned by 'healthy' people. Needless to say, temporal lobe epilepsy cannot explain an NDE precipitated by fear, depression, or isolation.

STIMULATION OF THE CORTEX

Debate relating to the role of the cerebral cortex in extraordinary experiences in our consciousness has been intensified by studies in which epileptic patients are subjected to electrical or magnetic stimulation of the cerebral cortex. We know that local electrical 'stimulation', which is usually applied during brain surgery, results in an inhibition or blockage rather than a stimulation of the 'stimulated' part of the cerebral cortex. This happens because the stimulation, like an epileptic seizure, wipes out the brain cells' local electromagnetic field. The effect depends on the duration and intensity of the electrical energy administered.

Some researchers claim that stimulation can trigger an out-of-body experience (OBE). Through local electrical stimulation of the temporal and parietal lobes during brain surgery for untreatable epilepsy, neurosurgeon Wilder Penfield (1955, 1958, 1975) occasionally managed to evoke memory flashes (never a life review), experiences of light, sound or music, dream-like experiences, and once an incipient OBE, during which a patient indicated 'Oh God! I am leaving my body'. Although he treated many hundreds of patients over the years, no real OBE with verifiable perception ever occurred and no transformation was ever reported. The effect of this stimulation was, in many respects, quite unlike an NDE.

In 2002 neurologist Olaf Blanke and others (2002) described a female patient with epilepsy who, after electrical stimulation (blockage), had an incomplete OBE with a distorted view of only her lower legs. The title of his article in *Nature* suggested that he had managed to locate the place in the brain where OBE originated. The article received extensive press coverage and caused quite a (premature) stir. In an article in 2004, Blanke produced another possible neurological explanation for out-of-body experiences (Blanke *et al.* 2004). He described six patients, of whom three had an atypical and incomplete OBE, that is without perception from the ceiling with verifiable elements of themselves or their surroundings; four patients with an autoscopy saw their own 'double' from the vantage point of their own body. In his article, Blanke describes an OBE as an 'illusion' caused by the temporary dysfunction or impairment of the temporal and/or parietal lobes. An illusion is an apparent reality or a false sense of reality, whereas an OBE involves a verifiable perception – from a position outside and above the body – of a resuscitation, traffic accident, or operation and of the surroundings in which these took place. An observation with verifiable aspects is, by definition, not an illusion.

As far as we are aware, none of the thousands of stimulated epilepsy patients around the world has ever reported a genuine OBE. The fact that in a single case, as described by Blanke, an abnormal bodily experience (illusion) was reported does not warrant comparison between this stimulated or impaired area in the brain of an epilepsy patient and the brains of normal individuals. Generalizing this finding seems more than unjustified given the fact that none of Blanke's small number of patients ever showed damage or dysfunction in exactly the same area. Therefore, we cannot cite the effect of stimulation of a certain area of an epilepsy patient's brain as evidence that this specific area actually causes the effect.

The Electroencephalogram (EEG) and sleep disorders as a result of an NDE

As part of a recent study among people who had an NDE in the past, an EEG was made during sleep (Britton and Bootzin 2004). An EEG registers electrical activity in the cortex. The REM (Rapid Eye Movement) phase is the phase in which people dream. Patients with an NDE were found to have fewer periods of REM sleep than a control group without an NDE. The EEG also detected anomalies in the left temporal lobe and symptoms of temporal lobe abnormalities such as unusual visual, auditory, or olfactory experiences but these are unlike the experiences that are reported during NDE. The NDErs also had a different pattern of sleep. However, the patients in this study were only studied *after* their NDE, which precludes a comparison with the EEG and sleep pattern *prior* to their experience.

Another study also reported REM sleep pathologies after an NDE (Nelson *et al.* 2006). This study examined the frequency of so-called REM intrusion. REM intrusion is accompanied by a sense of paralysis and confusing perceptions ('hallucinations') at the onset of sleep. The content of these perceptions do not resemble an NDE. A higher percentage of these symptoms (42%) were found in a self-selected group of people with an NDE in the past than in a control group which had been recruited among hospital staff and which reported a much lower percentage of REM abnormalities (7%) than is common among the general public (20 to 30%). The authors concluded that brain disorders that underpin REM intrusion may also precipitate NDE. The conclusion is, at best, premature, in part because the study was poorly designed, nearly 60 per cent did not report REM intrusion after an NDE, and patients were only examined after and not before their NDE (Long and Holden 2007). These studies therefore do not warrant any firm conclusions about either a neurological basis of an NDE or abnormal brain activity prior to an NDE. We can only conclude that compared to a control group without NDE, people with an NDE have a verifiably different sleep pattern, coupled with EEG anomalies in the temporal lobe. Perhaps the physical and psychological transformation after an NDE can shed a new light on the registered changes in electrical activity in the brain.

The Dutch study in survivors of cardiac arrest: A rebuttal

In order to obtain more reliable data to corroborate or refute the existing theories on the cause and content of an NDE, I felt we needed a properly designed scientific study. This was the reason why in 1988 my colleagues and I started a prospective study of 344 consecutive survivors of cardiac arrest in ten Dutch hospitals with the aim of investigating the frequency, the cause and the content of an NDE. We wanted to know if there could be a physiological, pharmacological, psychological or demographic explanation why people experience enhanced consciousness during a period of cardiac arrest. We studied patients who survived cardiac arrest, because this is a well-described life-threatening medical situation, which is also called 'clinical death'. These patients will ultimately die from irreversible damage to the brain if CPR is not initiated within five to ten minutes. It is the closest model of the process of dying.

The result of the study was that 18 per cent of the patients who survived cardiac arrest reported an NDE, and 82 per cent did not. But what could distinguish the small percentage of patients who report an NDE from those who do not? We found to our surprise that neither the duration of cardiac arrest (two minutes or eight minutes) nor the duration of unconsciousness (five minutes or three weeks in coma), nor the need for intubation in complicated CPR, nor induced cardiac arrest in electrophysiological stimulation (CPR within 30 seconds) had any influence on the frequency of NDE. Neither could we find any relationship between the frequency of NDE and administered drugs, fear of death before the arrest, nor foreknowledge of NDE, gender, religion or education.

Therefore, in our prospective study it is our contention that there were no physiological, pharmacological or psychological factors that caused these experiences during cardiac arrest. With a purely physiological explanation such as lack of oxygen in the brain most patients who had been clinically dead should report an NDE, because all patients in our study had been unconscious because of lack of oxygen in the brain resulting from their cardiac arrest (van Lommel et al. 2001). However, only 18 per cent reported an NDE. Our study showed clearly that during the period of unconsciousness due to a life-threatening crisis like cardiac arrest patients may report the paradoxical occurrence of enhanced consciousness experienced in a dimension without our conventional concept of time and space, with cognitive functions, with emotions, with self-identity, with memories from early childhood and sometimes with (extra-sensory) perception out and above their lifeless body (OBE).

Summary of physiological theories

Electrophysiological activity of the temporal lobes, anoxic brain damage, psychoactive biochemicals have all been implicated as possible causes of NDEs. However, while these explain certain aspects of the phenomena, none seem to be able to provide a unified theory that will explain the entirety of the experience. At various stages the described effects due to the above mentioned are not or not entirely consistent with the typical NDE elements, especially the most striking and distinctive elements such as out-of-body experiences with verifiable perception, a panoramic life review, an encounter with deceased persons, or a conscious return into the body. A reductionist approach will of necessity limit a more encompassing holistic view to the aetiology of NDEs. Further carefully designed research studies, with the daily advances of scientific knowledge, will assist in unravelling the mysteries of NDE.

Questions about the relationship between consciousness and the brain

Since the publication of four scientifically designed studies (Greyson 2003; van Lommel *et al.* 2001; Parnia *et al.* 2001; Sartori 2006) with a total of 562 survivors of cardiac arrest, with strikingly similar results and conclusions, the phenomenon of the NDE can no longer be scientifically ignored. It is an authentic experience, which cannot be simply reduced to imagination, fear of death, hallucination, psychosis, the use of drugs, or oxygen deficiency, and people appear to be permanently changed by an NDE during a cardiac arrest lasting only a few minutes. According to these studies, the current materialistic view of the relationship between the brain and consciousness held by most physicians, philosophers and psychologists is too restricted for a proper understanding of this phenomenon. There are now good reasons to assume that our consciousness does not always coincide with the functioning of our brain: enhanced consciousness can sometimes be experienced separate from the body.

With lack of evidence for any other theories for NDE, the concept thus far assumed but never scientifically proven, that consciousness and memories are produced by large groups of neurons and are localized in the brain should be discussed. How could a clear consciousness outside one's body be experienced at the moment that the brain no longer functions during a period of clinical death, even with a flat EEG? Such a brain would be roughly analogous to a computer with its power source unplugged and its circuits detached. It couldn't hallucinate; it couldn't do anything at all. Furthermore, even blind people have described veridical perceptions during OBE at the time of their NDE. Scientific study of NDE pushes us to the limits of our medical and neurophysiological ideas about the range of human consciousness and mind–brain relation.

Brain function during cardiac arrest

So we have come to the surprising conclusion that in our study during cardiac arrest NDE was experienced during a transient functional loss of all functions of the cortex and of the brainstem, with a flat-line EEG. And because of the occasional and verifiable out-of-body experiences we know that the NDE with all the reported elements must happen *during* the period of unconsciousness, and not in the first or last seconds of cardiac arrest. But how is it possible that a clear consciousness can be experienced outside one's body at the moment that the brain no longer functions, and how do we know that the EEG is flat in those patients with cardiac arrest, and how can we study this?

Through many studies with induced cardiac arrest in both human and animal models cerebral function has been shown to be severely compromised during cardiac arrest, with complete cessation of cerebral flow (Gopalan *et al.* 1999), causing sudden loss of consciousness and of all body reflexes. Also the abolition of brainstem activity with the loss of the gag reflex and of the corneal reflex, and fixed and dilated pupils are clinical findings in those patients (Parnia and Fenwick 2002). The function of the respiratory centre, located close to the brainstem, also fails, resulting in apnoea (Parnia and Fenwick 2002). The electrical activity in the cerebral cortex (but also in the deeper structures of the brain in animals shown by Branston *et al.* 1984) has been shown to be absent after 10–20 seconds (a flat-line EEG) (Clute and Levy 1990; Losasso *et al.* 1992; Mayer and Marx 1972; De Vries *et al.* 1998).

In acute myocardial infarction the duration of cardiac arrest in the Coronary Care Unit is usually 60–120 seconds, in an out-of-hospital arrest it even takes much longer. Therefore, all 562 survivors of cardiac arrest in the four aforementioned prospective studies must have had a flat EEG. The quite often proposed objection that a flat-line EEG does not rule out any brain activity, because it is mainly a registration of electrical activity of the cerebral cortex, misses the mark. The issue is not whether there is any brain activity of any kind whatsoever, but whether there is brain activity of the specific form regarded by contemporary neuroscience as the necessary condition for conscious experience, with visible and measurable simultaneous activities in many neural centres (Kelly and Kelly 2007). And it has been proven that there is no such specific brain activity at all during cardiac arrest. A flat-line EEG is also one of the major diagnostic tools for the diagnosis brain death, and in those cases the objection about not ruling out any brain activity whatsoever is never mentioned.

Pathophysiology and beyond

It is indeed a challenge to discuss new hypotheses that could explain the possibility to have clear and enhanced consciousness with memories, with self-identity, with cognition, with emotion, with the possibility of perception out and above the lifeless body, to explain the reported interconnectedness with the consciousness of other persons and of deceased relatives, to explain the possibility to experience instantaneously and simultaneously (non-locality)* a review and a preview of someone's life in a dimension without our conventional body-linked concept of time and space, where all past, present and future events exist, and even to explain the experience of the conscious return into the body. In my book (van Lommel 2010) I describe a concept in which our endless consciousness with declarative memories finds its origin in, and is stored in, a non-local space, and the brain only serves as a relay station for parts of this non-local consciousness to be received into or as our waking consciousness. Could our brain be compared to the TV set, which receives electromagnetic waves and transforms them into image and sound? Could it as well be compared to the TV camera, which transforms image and sound into electromagnetic waves? These waves hold the essence of all information, but are only perceivable by our senses through suitable

---

* Non-locality refers to a dimension where time and space play no role, where everything is instantaneously and continuously connected. (According to quantum physics non-local space represents a hidden reality that exerts a constant influence on our material world).

instruments like camera and TV set. The function of the brain could so be compared with a transceiver, a transmitter/receiver, or interface, quite like a computer that of course does not produce the internet with more than a billion websites, but only receives it. Different neuronal networks function as interface for different aspects of our consciousness, and the function of neuronal networks should be regarded as receivers and conveyors, not as retainers of consciousness and memories. In this concept, consciousness is not rooted in the measurable domain of physics, our manifest world. This also means that our endless or enhanced consciousness in non-local space is inherently not measurable by physical means, which could be compared with gravitational fields that are also not measurable but still continuously influence the whole universe. However, the physical aspects of consciousness, which originate from the wave aspect of our non-local consciousness through collapse of the wave function ('objective reduction') can be measured by means of neuro-imaging techniques like EEG, fMRI, and PET-scan ('neural correlates').

Conclusion

According to the aforementioned prospective studies in survivors of cardiac arrest, the current materialistic view of the relationship between the brain and consciousness held by most physicians, philosophers and psychologists is too restricted for a proper understanding of this phenomenon. With the concept of a non-local consciousness all reported elements of an NDE during cardiac arrest could be explained. I have come to the inevitable conclusion that most likely the brain must have a facilitating and not a producing function to experience consciousness. By making a scientific case for consciousness as a non-local and thus ubiquitous phenomenon I question a purely materialist paradigm in science.

CHAPTER 7

Psychological Aspects of Near-Death Experiences
SATWANT K. PASRICHA

Introduction

There is enough evidence to show that near-death experiences (NDEs) produce enduring psychological changes in the beliefs, values, attitudes and behaviour of near-death experiencers (NDErs)* (Flynn 1982; Gabbard and Twemlow 1984; Greyson and Stevenson 1980; Noyes 1980; Pasricha 1995, 2008; Ring 1980; Sabom 1982). Certain features of NDEs may resemble psychopathological conditions in their manifestation and may be mistakenly treated accordingly. Therefore adequate knowledge of NDEs is important for physicians and other health and mental health professionals (I shall also refer to them as clinicians) for making appropriate diagnosis or distinguishing NDEs from psychopathological states and offering suitable therapeutic interventions for which knowledge of different cultural beliefs regarding concepts of after-life is essential if one comes across cases from non-Western cultures.

---

* For convenience, I shall refer to NDEr as subjects or clients interchangeably and refer to all clients in the mascular gender without any gender bias.

Keeping the above in mind, I shall first summarize features of Indian cases. Next I shall briefly describe the psychological interpretations and psychopathological states that have been offered to explain NDEs, followed by the psychological sequalae of NDEs. In the last section, I shall enumerate a few points with suggestions that might be helpful to clinicians in helping NDErs who seek professional help.

Summary of Indian cases

Osis and Haraldsson (1977) conducted a survey of visions of 704 dying patients out of which 64 patients reported NDEs. We have investigated nearly 95 NDE cases in India, 67 of which I identified through the conduct of systematic surveys. I shall summarize features of Indian cases followed by three illustrative case reports from south India from my own records. For more such reports from south and north India see Pasricha (1995, 2008), and Pasricha and Stevenson (1986).

A majority of subjects of the Indian cases (81%) reported having gone to the other realms with the messengers of Yamaraj** or with deceased relatives. Nearly two-thirds of them reported having been passed to the man with a book and a mistake was discovered that they were taken there in place of another person or they were not yet scheduled to die, therefore, in spite of resistance on their part, they were sent back to earth with the remarks, 'You were not supposed to come here, another person had to come; you go back;' 'You are not the person who was sent for; you go back.' The mistake supposedly made by the messengers in bringing the subject is usually a small one. For example, the actual person who was supposed to have been brought had the same given name but belonged to a different caste or lived in a different but nearby village.

The subjects were brought back to the terrestrial life either by the same messengers or came back by themselves. Nearly half (47%) of them reported having been branded in the other realm and thus had residual marks following an NDE. The feature of residual marks is uncommon but not unknown. In the medieval literature, the marks after recovery from a near-death episode have been reported to occur on the shoulder and jaw of a saintly person which, according to him, had resulted from

---

** Yamaraj, the king of the dead, and his messengers, called Yamdoots, are well-known figures of Hindu mythology and current Hinduism. References to accounts of Yama or Yamaraj, Yamdoots and Chitragupt 'the man with a book' include Hazra (1940/1975), Moor (1809/1968), Walker (1968/1983), and Wilkins (1882/1978).

the fire of hell (Bede 1975). The residual marks, as we call them, are interpreted differently by the experiencers in northern and southern regions of India. As per the north Indian subjects these were generated as they were forcefully pushed down with an instrument, like a trident or a burning wood, when they resisted coming back from the other realm; on the other hand it is widely believed in southern India, that a mark is put on every person when he returns from the other realm to the terrestrial life. However, from the psychological point of view, these marks might have been generated due to autosuggestion or intense concentration on the event by the experiences as happens in the case of stigmatics.

I should also mention that some features like 'saw beings of light or religious figures', 'revived through the thought of the loved living persons', 'were sent back [from the other realm] by a loved one', and 'saw own physical body' while ostensibly dead, were not found in our initial study (Pasricha and Stevenson 1986) but were reported in the later studies (Pasricha 1993, 1995, 2008). So if these features are reported by an Indian subject in another culture they should not be considered as atypical features. However, none of our subjects had sensations of tunnels in any of our subsequent studies. Blackmore (1993) reported tunnel experiences in Indian population but her study had methodological and other flaws (Kellehear *et al.* 1994).

Case reports

CASE OF MRS V

At about the age of 36, Mrs V was very sick for about two to three months from fever, vomiting, loose motions, etc. She was not eating properly, she was malnourished, had become very weak and could not even speak. According to her son, one evening around 9 pm, she stopped talking and her body became cold. 'We were convinced that she was dead; we had even kept a lamp and lighted incense sticks near her body (a custom commonly observed near a dead body).' Next morning the family saw signs of life in her and heard her muttering, 'why did you come here; there is no place for you', which the family considered as 'loose talk'. Mrs V described her experience as:

> Dharamraja [Yamaraj] was sitting on a bison; he put a noose around my neck and pulled me up. He was black and fat and was wearing a huge crown. I saw oil was boiling there; two people would hold a sinner, one would cut him and push him into the boiling oil with huge rods. They were tied to

huge pillars. I could see my body lying here when my life was [being] taken. There was a bigger god, sitting on the throne. Some one was writing there. They said, 'you have no seat here' and I was sent back. Yamaraj brought me back on the bison and left me here.

Before the experiences she was weak and used to speak in a low tone, but that day (after NDE) she started talking loudly and was joyous.

CASE OF MR M

Mr M, at the age of 48, was suffering from typhoid. One morning when his family woke him up for coffee, he did not respond. They noticed that his breathing had stopped; the family took him as dead, and started preparing to perform for last rites. After about five hours, he stretched his right hand and his family noticed that he was breathing. Mr M gave the following account of his experience, which was corroborated by his son.

I was sleeping, one person came from the east; he had a rope in his hand. He asked me to go with him but I told him that I could not walk. He offered his hand to support me and said, 'I have been sent to take you; you have to come.' I walked with him and we reached a place that was not like earth; it was a flat land. We went near a gate; when I entered it, it was so bright there that I could not open my eyes for five minutes; I could not see anything for some time. The person who had brought me there took me to a place where a person was standing in front of a big book (of the size of a lorry). He looked into the book and said, 'You are not the person who was sent for, you go back.' I said that I was tired and could not walk to go back. He asked me to take some rest and then go. There I saw many people including some known persons from my village who had died earlier; they did not talk to me and continued to do their work. I did rest for some time and returned back with the same person.

Mr M became more religious and lost fear of death following the experience.

CASE OF MRS VN

At the age of 56, Mrs VN developed some skin problem under her thighs. One day she felt very tired; while talking to two persons she suddenly became unconscious and had the following experience:

Somebody came and took me to a place, which was like a big compound. My mother-in-law (who had died years ago) and another woman [from my village] called Munniamma, who had died of drowning, were sitting there. On the way I saw water everywhere and there was a path in between. There were 16 doors and there was a very bright light. Someone gave me a slip (entry pass). Then three or four persons took me to some place with the slip. There was one man who was sitting and writing about people. My slip was taken and given to him. When I was entering the door, they brought the slip back and asked me to go back. There was a man with a buffalo who asked the four men to send me away. I did not want to return so refused to come back. People were talking amongst themselves that a woman who gave birth to a child would come here. Then they placed something hot (cannot remember what it was) on my right forearm that caused a burn mark* and sent me back. There was a boil at that site when I regained consciousness. I heard afterwards that one woman died in another village after child birth.

Mrs VN said that she was glad to have gone away as she was fed up of suffering from the illness. She felt that she had done good deeds that are why she was sent back. There was no change in her attitude toward life in general but she has lost fear of death following the experience.

The above reports are presented essentially to illustrate features of Indian cases. The subjects had had their experiences several years earlier; so I did no therapeutic work with them. They all had initial confusion, bewilderment and emotional upheaval following NDE. With support from the family, community and their positive attitude, they were able to integrate their experiences, and were well adjusted.

Psychological interpretations of NDEs
Birth memory

The features of dark tunnel, bright light and going to another realm during NDEs have been psychoanalytically equated with remembering the process of birth by the experiencer (Sagan 1979). However, this

---

* She showed us a burn mark on her forearm, which she claimed had resulted from the burning in the other realm. There is a prevalent belief that branding is done in the other realm on people who are sent back.

theory has two important weaknesses. First, the experience of tunnels is absent in Indian cases (Kellehear *et al.* 1994; Pasricha 1995, 2008) or nearly absent in Thailand (Murphy 2001) and several other cultures (Kellehear 2008); or is not a common feature in many cases in cultures where it has been reported. Second, Blackmore (1983) reported that experiences of passing through a tunnel to another realm were also reported as frequently by persons born by caesarean sections as by persons born by normal vaginal delivery.

Although most studies have shown that NDErs are psychologically healthy individuals (Gabbard and Twemlow 1984; Irwin 1985; Locke and Schontz 1983), they have been mistakenly thought to have certain psychopathological conditions due to their phenomenological similarity in certain features. I shall briefly describe these conditions and mention points of differentiation from the NDErs.

Depersonalization

Depersonalization is an experience in which there is an alteration in body/mind perception. It is an experience in which the patient feels detached from experiences as if he were viewing them from a distance. Gabbard, Twelmow and Jones (1982) suggested differential diagnosis between OBEs and some psychological conditions, which are equally applicable to NDEs. Although both NDEs and depersonalization are precipitated by stress, they differ in the following ways.

The phenomenon of depersonalization occurs usually in the age range of 15–30, is more commonly reported among women, experienced as 'dream-like', characteristically unpleasant with an affect of anxiety, panic and emptiness, and serves a defensive purpose against life-threatening crisis (Noyes and Kletti 1976).

NDEs, on the other hand, have been reported in a wide range of age (2–65), with even sex-distribution; the observing self and functional self are experienced as one; NDEs are not experienced as dream-like; experiences are pleasant with pervasive feelings of calm, ecstasy, and peace; they do not seem to serve any obvious defence purpose.

Autoscopy

Autoscopy is an experience wherein a person sees his own self or his own double. The patient sees his image or apparition suddenly appearing in front of him. Since in out-of-body (OBE), as a feature of NDE, a person sees his own physical body before him, it has been confused for autoscopic phenomenon. The following will help in the differential diagnosis.

In the autoscopic phenomenon, the point of perception is not altered, the mind and the sense of self remain identified with the body; the patient sees his double which is perceived as an image of the self that generally imitates all the actions of the self; the double appears transparent and colourless. The affect is generally sad.

In contract, in the NDEs the mind is shifted from the body and sees his real body, which appears lifelike and lies inert; sadness of affect is rarely seen. Not all NDErs have an OBE.

Post-Traumatic Stress Disorder (PTSD)

Some NDErs appear distressed due to recurrent intrusive memories of the near-death event or due to difficulty in integrating the NDEs into their lives and this may resemble PTSD (Greyson 2001). They may evince decreased or no interest in day-to-day activities and face difficulty in maintaining relationships. However, the major point of differentiation from PSTD is that NDErs do not try to avoid frequent memories of NDEs and the positive affect decreases the possibility of subsequent stress symptoms.

Psychological sequalae of NDEs

Most experiencers report profound and long-lasting changes in attitudes, beliefs, values and behaviour as common psychological sequelae or after-effects of NDEs. The changes include enhanced self-confidence, self-esteem, compassion, generosity, feeling of contentment, increased interest in religiosity and/or spirituality, forgiveness, and detachment from worldly pleasures, reduction in unhealthy competitiveness, or needing approval of others, reduction in or loss of fear of death (Bauer 1985; Flynn 1982; Greyson 1983, 1992; Greyson and Stevenson 1980; Noyes 1980; Pasricha 1995, 2008; Ring 1980; Sabom 1982) leading to improved interpersonal relations and personal growth.

However, occasionally, negative psychological changes or effects have also been reported. These include increased fear of death and anxiety originating from witnessing hellish experiences, leading to difficulty in integrating such experiences in life (Greyson and Bush 1992; Pasricha 2008).

Suggestions for clinicians

Clinicians dealing with NDErs should have basic knowledge of NDEs regarding phenomenology and possible sequelae of NDEs for proper evaluation and choosing adequate therapeutic strategies for intervention. Most mental health professionals are trained in psychotherapeutic techniques but many are not sensitive to such unusual experiences as NDEs and so handle them inadequately by forcing a psychiatric diagnosis and (mis)treating them even with drugs which would cause more harm than do any good to the client. Therefore it is crucial for the clinicians to have a good understanding of NDEs and their components including paranormal and transcendental dimensions. It is also essential for them to be knowledgeable about beliefs and ideas associated with after-life among different cultures so that they can understand the experiences from the client's perspective. After having identified the NDEs, the next step is to provide counselling/psychotherapeutic support to the client and/or his family. Greyson (1997) found individual psychotherapy and group therapy quite effective with NDErs. One has to develop skills and sensitivity to accept and understand experiences of individual clients to provide adequate assistance.

There is no single therapeutic/counselling approach that can be suggested for dealing with NDEs. The best way to deal with them is to use an eclectic approach consisting of several techniques combined in which the clinician supports and guides the client in integrating NDEs.

Following general principles might be helpful to the clinicians.

- First of all the clinician should make the client comfortable. His first reaction to the client should be of a positive regard for both the client as well as his experiences. At no point should the clinician impose his personal beliefs or preconceived notions onto the client.

- The client should be assured of confidentiality, a basic element of all therapeutic relationships. The client should be assured that the information he provides will be kept confidential and not revealed to others without his informed consent.

- In a therapeutic alliance, the clinician should first allow the client to narrate his experience and then ask questions for clarification. In guiding the conversation the clinician should follow the client's account and understanding of the experience rather than judging experiences from his own perspective. Feedback in terms of the client's perceptions and emotions concerning the experience would be more helpful than offering interpretations which could prove counterproductive.

- The clinician should listen to the client attentively with no signs of disinterest or ridicule, either through words or gestures.

- Sharing experiences and associated emotions or confusion with a clinician or friend open to such experiences, and validation of his experiences against experiences of others, can prove cathartic or therapeutic and help him resolve distressing issues arising out of NDE. The clinician may communicate his reaction to the client, at the appropriate time, without challenging the client's perception of his experience. He should involve the client in finding solutions to his problems and guide him to come to terms with and integrating such experiences in day-to-day life.

- In my own experience with clients, I found a few (2–6) sessions were sufficient to reduce or eliminate distress and confusion following NDE. In one case the memories of the experience were interfering with the client's personal and professional life; and in the other case, the client was confused about the experience which he was not able to share with anyone.

- NDEs are sometimes reported to coexist with a pathological state and the two should be treated independently.

To sum up, NDEs usually occur to mentally healthy persons although their reactions may resemble pathological states. Therefore it is important that the clinician should be knowledgeable about phenomenology of both the NDEs and psychopathological states for adequate diagnosis; he should be equally conversant with the psychological changes that occur following NDEs and use appropriate intervention techniques. The clinician should have an unbiased approach to the client's experiences without imposing his own values or judgement on him.

CHAPTER 8

Light and Near-Death Experiences

ANTHONY PEAKE

A central factor in nearly all reported near-death experiences (NDEs) is the role of light. NDE survivors report a tunnel of light that takes them to a place bathed in a special form of light that does not hurt the eyes. When in this state they encounter beings of light and cities of light and most who return claim that they have become 'enlightened'. This theme is carried through into the titles of books written on the subject. These include *Lessons from the Light* by Kenneth Ring and Evelyn Elsaesser-Valarino (2000), *Beyond the Light* by P.M.H. Atwater (2009), *The Light Beyond* by Raymond Moody (1988) and *The Truth in the Light* by Peter and Elizabeth Fenwick (1995).

Indeed in their book the Fenwicks inform us that 72 per cent of their collected near-death accounts state that 'light was the predominant feature' (Fenwick and Fenwick 1995, p.58) whilst others were more specific in that they described how the illumination consisted of 'golden light' and 'bright luminous light' (Fenwick and Fenwick 1995, p.51).

In his book Raymond Moody describes the light in the NDE as 'unearthly', as 'white or clear' with an 'indescribable brilliance' that does 'not in any way' hurt the eyes (Moody 1975, p.58). One of his experiencers reported that the light was a 'crystal clear light, and illuminating white light. It was beautiful and so bright, so radiant, but it didn't hurt my eyes. It's not any kind of light you can describe on earth' (Moody 1975, p.63).

I have long been intrigued by the significance of this 'light experience' as part of the NDE. Indeed I am of the opinion that light is the major factor and a series of recent developments in neurology and quantum physics lead me to believe that we are on the verge of making a significant breakthrough that will finally present a scientifically viable explanation of this fascinating phenomenon.

In this chapter I will discuss the work of two Austrian researchers, Dr Engelbert Winkler and Dr Dirk Proeckl. I will then present my own model by which their work can be placed within a working theoretical model of consciousness.

The effects of light and the Elias Project

Dr Engelbert J. Winkler is a psychotherapist and clinical psychologist in Austria. His work is centred on clients who have severe psychological and social problems. In 1994 he founded a co-operative for crisis intervention, which initially was a counselling centre for children and teenagers with serious behavioural problems. Over time, the co-operative has expanded its services into the area of family crisis counselling using unconventional alternatives. A number of promising concepts and pilot projects have been put into practice and have developed into essential aspects of the Tyrol Youth Services Department (Department of Youth Services).

What stimulated Dr Winkler's pioneering approach was a particularly difficult case he encountered a few years ago. It involved a profoundly traumatized boy of nine years of age. This child had shown increasingly problematic behavioural problems since the suicide of his father some months before. Those responsible for the well-being of the boy had become particularly concerned when he had started to threaten suicide. For this reason they decided to approach Dr Winkler. Dr Winkler agreed and decided that the best approach would be to use a component crisis intervention programme that would use the theme of death and dying in a way appropriate for a child of this age.

Unfortunately these interventions did not have the desired effect. Indeed the child stated that he did not believe that he would survive to his next birthday, which was six months away. With mounting concerns Dr Winkler involved various family members in the therapy but as time progressed the boy lapsed deeper and deeper into a depressed state of mind.

Dr Winkler decided that a radical solution was required. As a member of the International Association of Near-Death Studies (IANDS), Dr Winkler knew of the seemingly therapeutic effect of the NDE. Indeed as an experiencer himself he was well aware of how the NDE can be a positive and life-enhancing experience, even with those who survive suicide attempts. His interest was such that he had met with many suicide survivors who had discovered, as one survivor put it, 'a beauty beyond any earthly ability to imagine'. Intriguingly, however, these individuals who previously had been pushed to such a state of despair that they wished to end their lives now approached life with great optimism and happiness. It was as if their 'glimpse' of the world beyond had given them a new appreciation of the beauty of life. These encounters had led him to the conclusion that maybe this could be applied in some way to his young patient.

However, in order to apply such a radical solution Winkler had to be sure that such an approach would work for a child of nine years of age. He devised an experiment with some local school children of a similar age to his patient. He wrote a short text, which he called 'The Day Elias Died'. This short piece of prose described a 'typical' NDE. This was then read to the children and, with the assistance of a local art teacher, the children were asked to draw a picture based upon the basic story. The results were amazing. As Winkler later wrote in a web article, 'The pictures they created gave me the impression that they still had some memories of that place to which we all must return to someday. Their pictures contained details which went beyond what I had included in the story' (Winkler undated).

Winkler then took the pictures to the home of his patient and, in the company of the child's mother and siblings, showed the drawings to the family. The result was astounding. His patient showed deep interest in the pictures and, with his siblings, discussed his favourite sections of the story. Soon he had created his own picture and he and his family were openly discussing the death of their father. Suddenly the child's suicidal comments ceased and he began to look forward to his birthday.

By applying the story 'The Day Elias Died' to other similar clients Winkler gradually came to the conclusion that by discussing and visualizing the classic light-related elements of the NDE scenario depressed patients can be given a whole new, and positive, viewpoint on life. This was to develop into something that Winkler called 'The Elias Project' and such was the success that he subsequently published a book,

The Occidental Book of Death and Dying, based upon this principle (Winkler 2007).

The simple visualizing of this 'light' was enough to engender a massively positive response in most of his clients. Furthermore Winkler discovered that this therapy could be considerably shortened. Indeed satisfactory results were also achieved for seemingly hopeless cases. He concluded that light, even the visualization of light, when envisaged within the context of the NDE, evoked some deep-rooted reaction that was, in all cases, therapeutically positive.

Winkler discussed these findings with his long-term associate Carola Proeckl. Carola suggested that it would be beneficial if he discussed the findings of the Elias Project with her husband, consultant neurologist Dr Dirk Proeckl. It was clear after the first meeting that Dr Proeckl was the ideal person to devise a neurological model by which the therapeutic power of light could be more effectively applied.

Taking advantage of the fact that key functional areas of the brain do not differentiate between imagination and real occurrences the two researchers started to work on a way in which external light could be used to reproduce the light experience as encountered in a near-death scenario.

They applied elements of two visual effects that are known to have direct neurological consequences that can be measured by using an electroencephalograph (EEG). These are known as the Visual Evoked Potential (VEP), (Regan 1989) and Flicker Fusion Threshold (FFT) (Hecht and Verrijp 1933).

By testing the electrical patterns in the brain as different combinations of VEP and FFT Winkler and Proeckl began to build up a neurological model of what were most effective in evoking altered states of consciousness similar to the NDE.

By placing sensors on the surface of the skull the two researchers were able to measure what is known as the Event-Related Potential (ERP) (Coles and Rugg 1996). In simple terms what is happening when an ERP is measured is that the researcher is, in effect, recording electrical activity of the brain, which could be linked to processing of thoughts and perceptions. In this way Winkler and Proeckl could objectively test the effectiveness of certain light sequences in generating specific ERP patterns.

Furthermore by meticulously testing combinations of light flickering at controlled speeds (stroboscopic) and additional combinations of white light of varying 'temperatures' Winkler and Proeckl were able to isolate a series of programmes that consistently brought about altered states. From this information they were able to design a light device that could be programmed to present varying degrees of altered states to the volunteers. The device is now known as the Lucid Light Device, affectionately called 'Lucia' (Winkler undated).

The final production model has a series of individual light bulbs, which produce plain white light with different 'temperatures'. White light comes in different forms, known as its 'colour temperature'. White light has a range of colours from one similar to normal incandescent bulbs to 'cool white' and 'cool daylight'. The actual temperatures of these white lights similarly range from 2700 degrees Kelvin to 6500 degrees Kelvin. These varying versions of white light bring about a flickering effect as well as a constant shining light.

Many volunteers have now experienced the effects of 'Lucia' (including the author of this article) and every single one has reported experiencing varying degrees of altered states of consciousness. However, Winkler and Proeckl were concerned that the device was generating these states in subjects who had nothing to compare them with. What they needed was a group of individuals who would be able to compare these artificially generated states with ones that had been produced naturally. Fortunately there is such a 'control' group, individuals trained in the fascinating technique of mind-control called 'Dream Yoga'.

Yoga and the light

Dream Yoga is a crucial element of an ancient Tibetan tradition known as Bön. Although part of the greater school of Tibetan Buddhism, Bön takes many of its techniques of spiritual enlightenment from the much older, shamanic, tradition of the Tibetan Plateau (Kvaerne 2001). Central to this tradition is the primacy of light in spiritual development. For the Bön the source of all consciousness is a multi-coloured sphere of light that exists outside of space and time. This source of 'enlightenment' can be accessed by deep meditation and by entering dream-states in which the 'Clear Light of Death' can be encountered.

In effect this Clear Light is the meditator's 'true self' and in merging with this light the meditator's soul can avoid the compulsory rebirth that is forced upon those who remain in the Bardo state* ignorant of its true purpose. In becoming a literal 'enlightened being' the soul remembers all its previous lives and can decide if it wishes to return to follow the cycle of birth and death again. Such enlightened beings are called 'Tulkas'.

A secondary light source is called the 'Clear Light of Sleep'. This can be encountered in the borderland between sleep and wakefulness. In Western psychological terminology this liminal state is called *hypnagogia* when encountered at the onset of sleep and *hypnapompia* when encountered on awakening (Mavromatis 2010). This is exactly the state of altered consciousness that Dr Winkler and Dr Proeckl believe is stimulated by their device.

In April 2010 Dr Winkler, Dr Proeckl, Carola Proeckl and Professor Erlendur Haraldsson of the University of Iceland travelled to Tibet to test the effectiveness of Lucia on a small group of individuals trained in Dream Yoga meditation techniques. The results were astonishing. One subject stated that it was like 'seeing a mandala with one's eyes shut'. Another, Buchung Changlochen, reported that the lamp made it possible for him to focus his spirit inward and cut out the outside world. He added that he felt that he had left his body behind and was in a state whereby he was surrounded by a light consisting of many vivid colours. The researchers were delighted that their neurological and psychological research was supported by such deeply meditative individuals.

Dr Winkler explained to me that 'Both the impressions of our testees and also old Tibetan learning support the thesis that the effect of Lucia can be directly compared to spiritual experiences. The hypnogogic light experience corresponds to experiences in deep meditation'.

It was clear from both the Dream Yoga and Bön tradition that light is of profound significance in the generation of internalized sensory experiences. Significantly in the Bön tradition the experience of enlightenment, as a non-dual source** of the consciousness of experience, corresponds to a multi-coloured sphere of light.

As scientists Proeckl and Winkler were interested to know exactly what is taking place within the brain when it is stimulated by 'Lucia'. What neurochemical process is involved and, more importantly, is there

---

*   According to Tibetan Buddhism the 'Bardo State' is a state of awareness that is experienced between the ending of one life and being reborn in another.

**   This is the belief that matter and mind are actually aspects of the same thing, in contrast to most Western philosophy which suggests that mind and matter are very different 'things'.

a specific location within the brain that is responsible for these altered states of consciousness?

Within two days a clue to the first question was to present itself.

On a visit to the palace of the Dalai Lama the team were to make an astounding discovery. In one of the rooms of this huge building they were shown a series of glass cases containing calcified natural history specimens. These large, pine-cone like structures were quickly recognized by the visitors. They were pineal glands, probably taken from the brains of long-dead elephants. On further questioning it was discovered that these objects are the subject of great veneration for members of the Bön tradition. These relics bore witness to the importance laid on this part of the brain as a central channel for spiritual experiences.

Was this the answer? Was this most mysterious of all the organs of the brain responsible for the internal generation of the lucid-light experience?

The pineal gland

This tiny reddish-grey object about the size of a grain of rice is found in all animals and because of its odd singularity has been an area of profound interest for hundreds, if not thousands, of years (Stehle *et al.* 2011). In shape it is reminiscent of a tiny pine cone. This led to it being called the 'pineal' gland. An earlier, and profoundly significant, name is the 'epiphysis' (from the Greek, *epi physis* to 'grow' or 'bring forth').

This singularity led ancient cultures to see it as an organ of significance. Many thought it to be the 'third eye', the place where the soul could look inwards into the worlds within as the eyes looked out at the world without (Stehle *et al.* 2011).

Interestingly modern scientific advances have shown that this organ not only lives up to its enigmatic reputation but also that the ancients had made surprisingly accurate observations about its function. For example, our advanced skills in medical dissection have shown that the front section of the pineal gland contains all the structures found in the human eye. It therefore should come as no surprise that research has shown that cold-blooded (poikilothermic) animals perceive light through their pineal gland. (Meissl and Yanez 1994; Stehle *et al.* 2011) This may be of significance with regard to human development. It has long been suggested that as the foetus develops within the womb it goes through its own mirror-image of evolution. It is logical to conclude that at some stage it will go through the poikilothermic stage. If this is the case then this should be when the pineal gland is also light sensitive and, in effect, is a genuine 'third eye'.

It is now known that the pineal gland has a crucial role in the generation of a chemical compound known as melatonin. Known as the 'hormone of darkness', this substance is secreted into the blood by the pineal gland as a way of telling the body that it is going dark and that the organism needs to sleep.

In order to facilitate this there has to be a mechanism whereby the pineal gland, buried deep within the skull, can differentiate between light and dark. Experiments have shown that the photoreceptors in the retina send a signal along the retinohypothalmic tract to the suprachiasmatic nucleus (SCN) and a similar signal follows a route along the upper thoracic spinal column to the superior cervical ganglion whose post-ganglionic sympathetic fibres innervate the pineal gland (Moller and Baeres 2002; Stehle *et al.* 2011). On receipt of this signal an enzyme known as serotonin-N-acetyltransferase (NAT) is released within the pineal gland, which, in turn, generates the production of melatonin (Pandi-Perumal *et al.* 2006; Stehle *et al.* 2011).

However, there is evidence that the light sensitivity of the pineal gland is looking for light from another source other than the retina. Vestigial Photoreciptivity within the pineal gland has been suggested by the discovery of pigmented cells arranged in a rosette-like structure reminiscent of developing retinal structures. This discovery suggests that human pineal glands exhibit transient cellular features reminiscent of developing photoreceptor cells as shown in other mammals. Furthermore in 1977 the light-sensitive compound phosphorus was discovered within the pineal gland (Vivien-Roels and Humbert 1977).

Thirty-seven years later, in 2007, an intriguing experiment took place at the National University in Taiwan: an experiment that suggested that maybe it is a different form of light that the pineal gland is designed to process, the light that is found in the often misunderstood word 'enlightenment'.

A small team led by Lyh-Horng Chen studied 20 subjects, 11 men and nine women, who practised the Chinese meditation technique known as 'Chinese original quiet sitting'.

The subjects volunteered to have their brains scanned using the medical process known as fMRI (functional magnetic resonance imaging). This measures the changes in blood flow within the brain and, in doing so, can show which parts of the brain are active when the subject is thinking about particular tasks or concepts. In other words it can measure 'thought'.

All the subjects were then asked to recite some of the traditional mantras that are used as part of this religious technique. By repeating these phrases the adherents claim to fall into deep meditative states similar to those experienced by the Tibetan Bön. Interestingly each subject showed increased activity in the pineal gland during these exercises. In a report in the UK magazine *New Scientist* Chen concluded 'There is no definition of "soul" in the scientific field. However, our results demonstrate a correlation between pineal activation and religious meditation which might have profound implications in the physiological understanding of mind, spirit and soul'(Chen 2007).

Here we have evidence that the pineal gland is of significance. However, such results tell us that something is happening but not what is happening within the pineal gland at these times and where the information is sourced to create these internal journeys to other states of awareness.

However, some interesting new developments in quantum physics may suggest some very exciting answers. Answers that may bring about a genuine paradigm shift in our understanding of the nature of consciousness itself.

Accessing memories

Western science is convinced that consciousness, or more specifically, self-aware consciousness, is a product of brain processing. The person reading these words is simply a collection of electrical charges 'manifesting' in the neurons the brain. However, as Australian philosopher David Chalmers has pointed out, this model has a huge problem. How can an amalgamation of inanimate molecules and similarly inanimate electrons bring about self-aware consciousness? How can 'manifest' particles create the non-manifest inner world of thoughts, dreams, ambitions and personality? He calls this the 'Hard Problem' and it is clear that our present paradigm simply cannot explain this mystery (Chalmers 1995).

However, recent discoveries have suggested that the brain is not merely a classical biochemical system but something far more complex; a 'macroscopic quantum system' that functions by drawing up information from a fascinating new form of energy known as 'Zero Point'. But what is even more pertinent in relation to the work of Winkler and Proeckl is that this energy manifests itself as light.

Zero Point Energy is a consequence of the Heisenberg Uncertainty Principle. This states that if we know the position of a sub-atomic particle we cannot know its speed and if we know its speed we cannot know its momentum. If a particle were at rest we would know both. Such particles can never be at rest, not even at absolute zero, the coldest state known to science. This is minus 273.15 degrees Celsius. This is three degrees below the temperature of the vacuum of space. Why this is of significance is that there should be no energy at absolute zero but there is. All space is filled with this quantum vacuum energy. It fills everything and in doing so changes what we think is a vacuum into a space absolutely full to the brim with energy. This energy exists, as all energy does, within a field. Not surprisingly this is called the 'Zero Point Field' or ZPF (Laszlo 2007).

This has interesting parallels with ancient Chinese philosophy that suggested that there is no such thing as empty space. For philosophers such as Chang Tsai the bedrock of reality is the *ch'i*. *Ch'i* translates as 'gas' or 'ether' and is a tenuous and non-perceptible form of matter, which is present throughout space and can condense into solid material objects.

The idea that matter somehow condenses out of the *ch'i* is amazingly prescient because there is a process that echoes perfectly this most ancient of ideas. This fascinating new form of matter is called Bose-Einstein Condensation and just like Chang Tsai suggests this is where the *ch'i* is seen to form a condensation out of the vacuum.

This new form of matter was first predicted by Indian physicist Satyendra Nath Bose, a scientist brought up within the Eastern rather than the Western philosophical tradition. In a paper that he sent to Albert Einstein in 1924 he described how it may be the case that if particles were cooled to a few degrees above absolute zero they may change from being a single particle to a collection of particles that act as if they were one (Bose 1924). Such a bizarre idea was proved when the first Bose-Einstein condensate was created in 1995 at the University of Colorado. Many years before, in 1938, a similar phenomenon was observed when a substance called helium 4 was found to have absolutely no viscosity. This meant that it could flow with absolutely no loss of energy (Steele 2009).

In principle what is happening is that all the particles within the condensate have become one, a single particle spread out in space and time. These condensates pull their energy directly out of the ZPF in the form of Zero Point Energy. Indeed many of us use a Bose Einstein condensate when we listen to music using a CD player. The information from the disc is read using a laser beam and a laser beam is technically coherent light – a beam in which all the light particles (photons) are sharing a single 'coherent' state. But there is another application of laser technology that has direct reference to the workings of the human brain, the hologram.

Holograms are three-dimensional images created by using lasers to 'photograph' an object and then reproducing the subsequent image by illuminating it with another set of lasers. This is again an application of coherent light in which a seemingly solid image can be reproduced from stored information. In 1986 two Japanese researchers, Isuki Hirano and Atsushi Hirai, suggested that coherent light is generated in vast quantities by tiny structures found deep within the neurons of the brain (Hirano and Hirai 1986). These structures, known as microtubules, are so small that it is possible that the energy they use to generate the coherent light is Zero Point Energy drawn directly from the ZPF. In other words they draw energy from what Indian traditional philosophy called the 'Akashic Record' and what Chang Tsai knew as the *Ch'i*.

If Hirano and Hirai are correct then the Akashic data can be reassembled using the laser-like coherent light to create seemingly three-dimensional holographic images of the stored information. This would create in the mind of the experiencer a three-dimensional version of the recording that would be totally lifelike in every way. It would be like the illusionary world of the *Matrix* movies. It would be indistinguishable from the 'real' thing. I use the speech marks because such a model suggests that the 'reality' we take for granted that is external to our bodies and supplied to us by our senses may not be as 'real' as we believe. Indeed modern neurology tells us that what we take to be external reality is a construct of the brain modelled out of the electro-chemical information supplied to it from our senses.

The question is: is there a portal within the brain whereby the riches of the Akashic Record can be accessed? Recent discoveries have suggested that an intriguing hallucinogenic substance may be excreted by the pineal gland. If this is the case then the body itself creates the neurochemical circumstances whereby consciousness can delve deeply into its own 'inner space' and there encounter a reality wrapped within a greater reality.

In order to appreciate how this process works we need to understand how the brain sends messages from one cell to another using a collection of fascinating chemicals called neurotransmitters.

Chemical messengers (the neurotransmitters)

Neurotransmitters are released by a neuron (brain) cell to stimulate other neurons in its vicinity and in the process transmit impulses from one cell to the other. In turn this facilitates the transfer of messages throughout the whole nervous system. The site where neurons meet is called the synapse, which consists of the axon terminal (transmitting end) of one cell and the dendrite (receiving end) of the next. A microscopic gap called a synaptic cleft exists between the two neurons. When a nerve impulse arrives at the axon terminal of one cell a chemical substance is released through the membrane close to the synapse. This substance then travels across the gap in a matter of milliseconds to arrive at the postsynaptic membrane of the adjoining neuron. This chemical release is stimulated by the electrical activity of the cell. Across the other side of the cleft, at the end of the receiving dendrite, are specialized areas that act as docking areas for particular neurotransmitters. These are known as 'receptors'. It is useful to visualize the receptors to be like docks at a port. Sometimes they will be open, letting in ships containing cargo and, sometimes, they will be closed and the ships cannot unload their goods (Stahl 2000).

If the newly arrived neurotransmitter chemical is allowed into the dock it is free to 'instruct' the dendrite to send a particular signal along to its nucleus then out to its own axons. When it does this it is said to be excitatory. Sometimes the effect of the neurotransmitter(s) released by the pre-synaptic axon is to inhibit rather than excite the post-synaptic dendrite. In this case it is said to be inhibitory (Stahl 2000).

Since their first discovery in the 1930s 50 or so neurotransmitters have been found, the most important being serotonin, noradrenaline, glutamate and a group of pain-killing opiates called endorphins. However one internally generated substance was to remain a mystery. However in 1972 Nobel-Prize winning chemist Julius Axelrod made a very surprising discovery.

In a routine test of some brain material Axelrod found traces of a substance known as dimethyltryptamine. Known as DMT this chemical is a member of the amine family. Seven years earlier another amine had been found in human blood. This was, in itself, a surprise as up until then amines had only been found in the cells of invertebrates. The discovery of an amine in the brain was a total puzzle. It was believed that these chemicals had no function within the human body. So why was DMT in the brain?

The mysterious function of amines within the body was further brought into question in 2001 when a new family of receptor cells was discovered. Called Trace Amine-Associated Receptors (TAARs) these cells were like locks in which only one key could be used, and that key was an amine. What this suggested was stunning, that amines are a form of neurotransmitter (Liberles 2009). As DMT is a form of amine then its reason for being in the brain was clear; DMT exists in the brain because the brain is designed to work with it.

DMT is known to be the most powerful hallucinogenic substance yet discovered. For centuries it has been used by shamans as a way to communicate with the 'upper' and 'lower' worlds. But now, it seems, neurologists have discovered that the brain may generate it naturally, that DMT is a natural element of how the brain functions.

Some scientists believe that there is one specific place in the brain that DMT is produced – the pineal gland. Indeed researcher Dr Rick Strassman of the University of New Mexico has further suggested that DMT may be responsible for the NDE itself (Strassman 2001).

And DMT is the substance that Winkler and Proeckl believe is responsible for the altered states of consciousness described by all who have experienced the Lucid Light Device. Could this be the link that has been long searched for that the light experience reported by virtually all who have reported an NDE is generated by the release of DMT within the brain? If so, how may this work?

An explanatory model of NDE

Earlier we saw how it may be possible for consciousness to access information directly from the Zero Point Field, also known as the Akashic Record or simply *ch'i*. The energy contained within this field, Zero Point Energy, can be perceived as light in the same way as electromagnetic energy is similarly perceived. We know from the work of Winkler and Proeckl that the stimulation of the pineal gland by the modulated light of Lucia can generate within the 'mind's eye' an 'inner light' of profound intensity. This echoes the beliefs of the Dream Yoga and Bön traditions who know this inner light as the 'Clear Light of Death'.

Could it be that the facilitator of this 'inner light' may be an internally generated version of DMT? There is sufficient evidence for researchers to pursue this possibility through empirical research. If DMT is subsequently found to have a crucial involvement in the workings of the brain then we may have the start of a working model of how consciousness can perceive two forms of light: the light of our everyday waking world that illuminates everything we see, and an inner light that is drawn up from the depths of the quantum world and illuminates our own inner universe.

If this is the case then we have, at last, a potential explanation for NDEs, out-of-the-body experiences, lucid dreaming and other 'altered states of consciousness'.

However, in presenting this model we end up with another, even greater question; which of these two 'illuminated' realities is real and which one is an illusion? Or are they both aspects of a greater reality?

CHAPTER 9

Religious Significance of Near-Death Experiences

PAUL BADHAM

Near-death experiences (NDEs) are important for religion because they appear to offer support for the claim that to die is not simply to 'expire' (i.e. to breathe out for the last time) but might better be described as 'the parting of soul and body'. Dr Gregory Shushan suggests that NDEs may be the source of such beliefs. He shows that in widely separated cultures (Ancient Egypt and Mesopotamia, Vedic India, Pre-Buddhist China, and Pre-conquest Meso-America) there are some commonalities in after-life beliefs, which suggest a shared origin in NDEs (Shushan 2009). The same also seems true in other religious traditions.

Early Israelite religion is unusual in that it had no real concept of the soul (Badham 1976) but in subsequent Jewish thought belief in the soul's immortality became a central belief (Cohn-Sherbok 1987). It is interesting to speculate what brought about that change. In an early Jewish mystical text called the *Zohar* we read: 'We have learned that at the hour of a man's departure from the world, his father and relatives gather round him and he sees and recognises them and they accompany his soul to the place where it is to abide' (*Zohar*, Vol. 2, p.307, see Cox-Chapman 1996, p.139). The question arises, how did they 'learn' this? One possible answer might be from reported NDEs. Modern NDE experiencers frequently report precisely such 'meetings' with deceased relatives and therefore an early NDE account may have been the source of this 'learning'.

Likewise the claim by many near-death experiencers to observe the way the people gather round the apparently dead body also corresponds to claims in religious tradition that immediately after death people are aware of the distress of their loved ones. For example, in *The Tibetan Book of the Dead* we read that when the person's 'consciousness-principle' gets outside its body 'he sees his relatives and friends gathered round weeping and watches as they remove the clothes from the body or take away the bed' (Evans-Wentz 1957, p.101).

In Zoroastrianism, it is intriguing that the name of their deity, 'Ahura Mazda' literally means 'The Being of Light'. This almost inevitably suggests that something akin to an NDE gave rise to this tradition. In Greek thought Plato played a key role in establishing the idea of the immortality of the soul and in his book, the *Republic*, says that the source of his belief was a story he had been told of a soldier called Er who was thought to have been killed in battle but who just before his cremation had 'come back to life and told the story of what he had seen in the other world' (Plato 1955, p.394).

Within Christianity the peak of mystical experience has always been described in terms of 'ecstasy', which literally means 'out-of-the body'. When St Paul found his religious authority challenged by the Corinthians he rested his claim to their respect explicitly on an experience, which reads very much like a contemporary NDE.

> I know a Christian man who fourteen years ago (whether in the body or out of the body I do not know God knows) was caught up as far as the third heaven. And I know that this same man (whether in the body or apart from the body I do not know God knows) was caught up into paradise, and heard words so secret that human lips may not repeat them. About such a man I am ready to boast. (2 Corinthians 12: verses 1–5)

St Paul was speaking autobiographically here as a few verses later he laments that 'to keep me from being unduly elated by the magnificence of such revelations I was given a thorn in the flesh...to keep me from being too elated' (2 Corinthians 12: verse 7). St Paul's experience included out-of-the-body experiences and visions of paradise, both of which are key features of the NDE

Commenting on these verses, St John of the Cross, the great 16th-century mystic, remarked that such experiences normally only occur when the soul 'goes forth from the flesh and departs this mortal life'. But in St Paul's case he was allowed these visions by special grace. Such visions however occur 'very rarely and to very few for God works such things only in those who are very strong in the spirit and in the law of God' (St John of the Cross 1957, p.84). St John of the Cross almost certainly had a comparable experience himself as evidenced by his poems where he speaks of 'living without inhabiting himself', 'dying yet I do not die' and as 'soaring to the heavens' (St John of the Cross 1960).

In Islam it is clear that a strong ecstatic element was present in all Muhammad's revelatory experiences. In one of his 'hadith' he claimed, 'Never once did I have a revelation without feeling that my soul was being torn away from me' (Armstrong 1993). More significantly his 'Night Journey' in which he ascended through the seven heavens has been interpreted in the Sufi tradition as an 'annihilation' (fana) followed by 'revival' (baqa) in which Muhammad passed through death to the vision of God, and was then restored to life with a greatly enhanced spirituality (Armstrong 1991, p.93). Rimpoche (1992) likewise notes that in Tibetan Buddhism NDEs have long been acknowledged as religiously significant in that 'returnees from death', *deloks*, have for centuries been regarded as important witnesses concerning the reality of the next world (pp.330–336).

During an NDE some report seeing a review of the their past life and many experience a range of mental images. This has led to the suggestion that the next stage of existence could be a mind-dependent world. H.H. Price, a former Professor of Logic at Oxford University, has spelt out how useful a mind-dependent world could be for reflection, recollection and reformation before moving on to a further stage of existence. This idea has been developed by John Hick who suggests that many lives in many worlds with intervals for reflection in between could be a way in which we could grow and develop after death (Hick 1976, p.270). He suggests that such a view would seem a natural development of Hindu concepts of the after-life which teach that at death we initially enter a world of desire (*Kama Loka*) (Hick 1983, p.120). This is understood as a mind-dependent state reflecting our memories and desires in which we stay before moving on to a new birth. Similar ideas seem present in *The Tibetan Book of the Dead* which speaks of the dying person seeing the radiant, pure and immutable light of Amida Buddha before passing into what is explicitly described as a world of mental images. Therefore NDEs appear to offer support for ideas present in both Hindu and Buddhist speculations concerning a future life and which also attune well with some contemporary Western hypotheses concerning the nature of the next stage of existence.

One feature of NDEs is the fact that 72 per cent of contemporary near-death experiencers report seeing a radiant light which they often describe as a loving presence and sometimes name in accordance with a religious figure from their own traditions. *The Tibetan Book of the Dead* speaks of the dying person seeing the radiant, pure and immutable light of Amida Buddha. But it also recognizes that people of other traditions will see and name it in accordance with their own religious beliefs. Thus the *Tibetan Book of the Dead* says 'The *Dharmakaya* (deity) of clear light will appear in whatever shape will benefit all beings'. Commenting on this verse for his English translation Lama Kazi Dawa-Samdup says:

> To appeal to a Shaivite devotee, the form of Shiva is assumed; to a Buddhist the form of the Buddha; to a Christian, the form of Jesus; to a Muslim the form of the Prophet; and so for other religious devotees; and for all manner and conditions of mankind a form appropriate to the occasion. (Evans-Wentz 1957, p.98)

Such an hypothesis seems a brilliant way of reconciling the fact that while people of a wide variety of traditions appear to have very similar experiences of encountering a being of light they each name it in accord with their own religious background. This is even true of atheists. When one very prominent 20th century atheist philosopher A.J. Ayer had an NDE he said afterwards 'I realized the light was responsible for the government of the Universe'. He also said 'on the face of it this experience is rather strong evidence for life after death'. Later he retracted his claim saying it had 'only slightly weakened' his belief that death would be the end but he continued to hope it would be (Ayer 1988). However, the fact that the NDE had so powerful an initial impact on a life-long atheist is highly significant.

Many resuscitated people speak of seeing and being welcomed into the world beyond by this wonderful and gracious 'Being of Light'. They often claim that this being knows them completely and has limitless compassion to them in welcoming them into the life beyond. It is interesting that this is remarkably like what the Pure-land scriptures say for they say that 'The Buddha of Infinite Light and Boundless Life' (*Amida*) has vowed to appear at the moment of death. Consequently when people 'come to the end of life they will be met by Amida Buddha and the Bodhisattvas of Compassion and Wisdom and will be led by them into Buddha's Land' (Bukyo Dendo Kyokai 1980, p.218). This combination of radiant light, wisdom and compassion correspond precisely to the descriptions given by the resuscitated of their experience of this encounter.

From a Catholic perspective the evidence from NDEs is very important. We have already noted that the great Christian mystics speak of religious ecstasy which literally means 'being taken out of one's body' and we saw how important this was both to St Paul and St John of the Cross. Similarly Catholic tradition as in the Dream of Gerontius has spoken of how angels of light will receive us at death. Heavenly visions always associated God with radiant light and traditionally saints are painted surrounded by a halo of light. Likewise 'seeing the light' has long been a metaphor for religious conversion. It is also a vital part of Catholic doctrine that we are both material and spiritual beings and that we can have religious experiences which transcend our bodily senses. As St Paul declared 'Spiritual things are spiritually discerned.' Most importantly of all the immortality of the soul is vital to Christian belief in life after death because it forms the bridge between this world and the unimaginably different resurrection life in heaven. According to the Papal Encyclical Man's *Condition After Death*,

> the Church affirms that a spiritual element survives and subsists after death, an element endowed with consciousness and will, so that the human self subsists, though deprived for the present of its complement of the body. To designate this element the Church uses the word 'soul' the accepted usage in Scripture and Tradition. (Neuner and Dupuis 1983, p.691)

It seems to me utterly remarkable that so often Western people who have an NDE describe being greeted into the life beyond by a being of radiant light with limitless compassion and understanding. The Pure-land scriptures are largely unknown among the general public in the West. So there can be no question of the experience being generated by expectation of such an outcome. On the other hand if the experiences that people have are accepted as genuine then this could be evidence that human destiny may indeed continue through death into another mode of life.

CHAPTER 10

Assessment and Management of Near-Death Experiences

PETER FENWICK

Near-death experiences (NDEs) have become part of our understanding of those abnormal mental states, which are associated with life-threatening crises. The phenomenology of these experiences is now well understood at a popular level, but although there is considerable research into the consequences of these experiences, these are not so well known to the medical community. This article looks briefly at the medical consequences of having an NDE and the psychological changes which often follow it. Briefly discussed are the mental states of the dying and the importance of these states for the relatives of the dying and their grieving.

Outcome of adult NDEs

NDE can occur as a result of any severe physical or surgical event which has brought the patient near to death, such as cardiac arrest, accidents, childbirth with haemorrhage. But it is important to recognize that experiences with similar phenomenology can also arise in quite different circumstances, when the subject is in fact not near-death at all. These have a psychological and not an organic cause and usually occur when the person is under great stress or intensely fearful – the so called 'fear death' experiences. A third group, again with similar phenomena, are the transcendent experiences which arise spontaneously, and it has been argued that these transcendent mystical experiences even if they have the same phenomenology should not be included in the NDE category (Fenwick and Fenwick 1995). The standard questionnaire for assessing whether an experience is a true NDE is its score on the Greyson NDE Scale (Greyson 1983) (see Appendix 3).

The outcome of an NDE will depend on its cause and whether or not there is associated brain damage. If the cause is organic, then brain damage is a possibility, which should always be considered and investigated. Psychological outcomes are classified by rating a questionnaire, the most commonly used of which is 'The Life Change Questionnaire', an instrument introduced by Greyson and Ring (2004). The questionnaire defines various psychological dimensions, for example self-confidence, fear of death, effect on spiritual development, and on social and personal relationships.

The changes found are an increased focus on the present, a deepening of religious faith and heightened spirituality. The most common reaction to the experience is loss of the fear of death with a strengthened belief in an after-life. Those who have had it tend to value life more highly and have a greater appreciation of the world around them. Because the experience is so overwhelming they feel compelled to find out more about it and its significance. They tend to become more socially conscious with a desire to serve society, show less inhibition about expressing emotions, and have increased compassion and love for others. Accompanying this is a reduction in drive for material gain or social position. Often they have a new sense of purpose and some come back saying they have a special mission to accomplish although they may not always remember just what this is (Noyes et al. 2009).

It must not be forgotten that many of the changes described above are also described in anyone who has come close to death, particularly cardiac arrest patients. Coming close to death leads to a re-evaluation of your personal life values, and also a renewed appreciation of life. It is thus not surprising that these changes are observed, although not as intensely in those survivors who did not have an NDE. An additional difficulty is that the organic factors due to changes in brain function have seldom been adequately examined and thus changes reported may have an organic cause rather than being due to the NDE. However, comparison of changes in people who have been near to death and have had an NDE with a control group who have also been near to death but have not had an NDE suggest that those who have not had an NDE have almost the same range of psychological changes as those who have one but the changes are not so marked (van Lommel *et al.* 2001).

Although the effects of the NDE are usually positive, a few people do report more negative effects. There are case reports of individuals who on recovering from the event can no longer tolerate the thought of living in this world. They feel bereft and long to get back to the very strong positive feelings of the NDE. They may become depressed or even actively suicidal. In another of the author's cases a patient required hospitalization for a number of months before she could fully integrate the powerful NDE experience and was able to return safely to her normal life. A small number of NDErs report that they relive the experience and this is not always welcome because it is so intense.

Hellish or negative NDEs

Negative NDEs are reported, though they are much less common. It is important to differentiate the true negative NDE from an intensive care psychosis. In the case of an NDE feelings of intense loneliness and abandonment seem to predominate. In an intensive care psychosis the patient will have the experience in a confusional setting and will from time to time partially regain clearer consciousness. Some report intense paranoid hallucinations and a common theme is that either devils or other people are setting out to kill them. As the patient improves and the psychosis clears the experience is seen to have been built on the sounds and sensations of the nursing procedures in the ICU (Greyson and Bush 1992).

Parapsychological phenomena

Clairvoyance, telepathy, out-of-body experiences, precognition and claimed healing ability are all reported sequelae of the NDE. There are case reports of patients finding some of these new sensitivities difficult

to live with. Intuition about negative happenings to family acquaintances is one, which is often quoted. Some NDErs no longer wear watches, because they frequently stop; they also report that complex electronic equipment tends to go wrong in their presence (Sutherland 1989).

Personality factors

There is a small literature on personality traits of people who have had an NDE. A tendency to dissociate is one such trait, and this is certainly characteristic of people who have out-of-body experiences. There is also some suggestion that NDErs have higher absorption scores (a tendency to focus on sensation) than those who had simple out-of-body experiences (Twemlow and Gabbard 1984–85). However, these are all post-hoc studies so it is not possible to know if the tendency to dissociate or show high absorption followed or preceded the NDE.

The aftermath

People's view of their NDE changes as time passes. Immediately after the experience the individual is frequently confused and has difficulty in slotting it into their usual world view. After such a strong emotional experience they have heightened sensitivity, and feel a loss of spatial boundaries and detachment from the everyday world. The experience may also flash back into consciousness.

As time goes on, some integration of the NDE into everyday experience occurs. Sometimes it is interpreted as a dream although some people hold it as an important transcendental experience. If, when they discuss it with medical personnel or their relatives, the experience is dismissed or negated, then they may not talk of it again for many years. If they feel unable to discuss what is to them a very meaningful experience they may be left with the feeling that they are in some way abnormal. If they meet a more helpful attitude then integration of the experience takes place more quickly.

Many experiencers feel they want to learn as much as they can about the experience and this information is now available through the internet. They may also seek validation through health care professionals who must be careful not to dismiss this important experience. Sutherland (1992) has described the stages through which people may pass in

assimilating the experience – blocked, arrested, steady and accelerated. A blocked experience is one which is thought by the experiencer to be meaningless and this view is reinforced by others who discount it. An arrested experience is one in which the person has started the integration process but without friends and professional support is unable to take it further. The other two stages are a continuing progression to a more integrated experience, and there is some suggestion that people who have had very profound and meaningful NDEs may do this more easily. Other authors have used slightly different schemes but essentially they are the same as that of Sutherland.

A study of suicide has compared those who had an NDE during their suicide attempt and those who did not. Those who had the positive experience of an NDE were found to have less suicidal ideation afterwards and to be much less likely to make a subsequent suicide attempt (Greyson 1992–93).

Treatment

If a patient has had an NDE then it may be important to investigate any features of brain damage as there is a correlation between those factors, which may result in an NDE, for example cardiac arrest or severe head trauma, and the occurrence of cerebral damage. MRI scanning for structural brain damage, EEG for abnormal electrical discharges and a full neuropsychological assessment to estimate cognitive function may all be necessary in order to get a reliable estimate of brain damage.

Immediately after an NDE the patient is often confused and unable to make sense of what has happened. It is helpful if they are encouraged to talk about the experience and reassured that they are normal and that over 10 per cent of the population has such experiences. As they come to accept this view they will probably want to know more about NDEs, and particularly why they should have had one. Should family members negate the experience or assume that the person who has had it is unbalanced, joint counselling may be helpful. It is also helpful if the person can be directed to an NDE support group where they can meet others who have had the experience. With adequate support it is unlikely that the NDEr will become depressed and withdrawn.

End-of-life experiences

Until recently there has been little research into end-of-life experiences. Studies in hospices have shown that in the two to three weeks before death a number of patients experience visions, usually of dead relatives. The patient usually says that the visitor has promised that they are going to come and accompany the dying on their journey, occasionally even giving a date for their return. These visions are comforting to the dying, who seem to lose any fear of death, and usually also to the relatives. Even if the dying person is unable to speak, their behaviour often suggests that they are seeing something or someone to whom they respond with joy. The research that has been done suggests that these visions are not due to medication or to confusional states of the dying. Neither do they seem to be linked to religious belief, desire for comfort or expectation (Fenwick and Fenwick 2008).

Just before death a number of the dying seem to transit between two different realms. They describe being in the hospice one moment and then in a transcendent reality, not unlike that described in the NDE, the next. Another phenomena sometimes reported by friends or relatives of the dying person is the 'death-bed coincidence' in which at the moment of death the dying person may appear to someone with whom they are closely emotionally connected, usually another family member. If the death occurs during the day the waking relative will describe a strong emotional feeling, sometimes non-specific, sometimes specifically of the person's presence, often with the feeling that they are in trouble. If they are asleep the dying person comes to them in a dream, in which they are often given the message that the person has died but is all right.

Other phenomena linked to the time of death, such as shapes seen leaving the body or light surrounding it, are also reported by carers and relatives of the dying and are usually interpreted by the relatives as an indication that some essence of the person has survived, and these too act as a source of comfort (Fenwick, Lovelace and Brayne 2009).

Treatment

End-of-life phenomena are relatively common although their exact incidence is not known and little research has been done. However, the accounts that are given show the importance of validation of these occurrences by carers and especially the medical profession. They help the family to grieve and are usually interpreted as a message about the continuation of personal consciousness of someone they love.

Prospecting in the Light

The Future of Near-Death Experiences Research

DAVID J. WILDE AND
CRAIG D. MURRAY

In the penultimate section of this book the task falls to the authors
to try to create a nexus between previous research findings and what
investigative developments and pathways might lie ahead. To date, much
of the research conducted on near-death experiences (NDEs) has been
focused on issues concerning either the veridicality of the phenomena,
or to more specifically determine the underlying processes by which the
phenomenon manifests itself. In reviewing the work presented thus far,
we believe there are numerous practical, theoretical and methodological
advancements that may form the basis of an exciting, broad-based
research agenda for the future.

In presenting our suggestions, though, we have opted to focus
on three broad areas of research whose findings we feel may resonate
with the kinds of questions clinicians, experients and interested lay
people ask. Mostly everyone we suppose would want to know if the
NDE really is a glimpse into the after-life or something far less esoteric.
Clinicians will likely want more knowledge they can usefully apply in

their everyday practice, for example, evidence regarding epidemiology, etiology, diagnositic criteria, any underlying pathologies, the longer-term response to the experience, and what therapeutic interventions one might fruitfully employ to deal with any related co-morbidities. Whereas, experients will doubtless be left with many questions centred on the meaning and sense-making of their experience. However, we feel we must begin our deliberations as all systematic researchers do, with basic definitions and theory.

Before undertaking any research, a researcher should have a clear and widely accepted definition of what it is they are investigating. Alas, for the NDE researcher there remains a general lack of agreement as to how best to define the phenomenon. This lack of accord has been highlighted by long-standing NDE researcher Bruce Greyson (2000) as a fundamental imposition towards developing the 'precision and credibility of near-death research' (p.342). In the same review, Greyson noted that, despite the development of a plethora of theoretical models proposing to explain the NDE – for example, Moody's (1975, 1977) original phenomenological model, Noyes (1972) developmental model, Lundahl's (1993) stage model and Greyson's (1983) own factor analytically derived model – none have been empirically tested to evaluate their clinical applications or predictive legitimacy. These are serious shortcomings indeed. Without a commonly agreed-upon definition of the NDE, findings from different studies remain closed to comparative evaluation. Theoretical models can only be developed or discounted as the empirically derived data for or against them accumulates. Without a foundation of reliable and valid research evidence, these models are little better than intellectual road maps that, whilst whetting academic appetites, are leading us virtually nowhere in terms of pragmatics. If NDE research is to continue, flourish, and more importantly, be accepted by the wider medical and scientific community, these basic issues must be addressed.

Despite the numerous NDE surveys that have been carried out, there remains a dearth of epidemiological data regarding NDE occurrence. As far as the authors are aware, only one nationally representative survey has been conducted by Perera, Padmasekara and Belanti (2005) in Australia. Whilst other surveys have been carried out, most of them have been inconsistent in the sample sizes they include and in their methods of data collection. Whilst the authors are not against research with small samples – there are certain desirable advantages in conducting such focused work, as we discuss later – the cornerstone of the survey method requires large, representative samples drawn from the general population in order to make an accurate statement regarding the true incidence of the NDE. Clinicians used to working in an evidence-based environment may find the paucity of such basic data frustrating. Epidemiological data is crucial as without it the clinician is left with a weak global context within which to evaluate the report of an NDE from a patient. Looking beyond the population in general to more specific sub-groups, more research should be focused on more precisely determining the prevalence of NDEs amongst children, the elderly, as well as members of various ethnic and religious groups.

One of the most enduring questions humankind has ever asked must surely be 'what happens when we die?' If taken at face value, the NDE might seem to be one of our best hopes of answering that question. Almost certainly many experients would probably agree. Yet, as John Palmer (2010) has recently written there is no consensus amongst parapsychologists regarding the survivalist issue. It is an intellectually and often emotionally polarizing debate, which we do not intend to get into here. Interested readers are thus directed to the following literature: Braithwaite (2008), Fenwick and Fenwick (1995), Murray (2010, Chapters 11 and 13) and Sartori (2008).

However, in pointing out the apparent discord in the scientific discourse regarding NDE veridicality, Palmer also noted that there is a fundamental question that many in the scientific community do agree would lead us in the direction of that answer, and that question is, when exactly does an NDE occur? At the risk of stating the obvious, it is a very challenging question and a definitive answer is still a very long way off using even the most advanced research methods and technology. The assumption by pro-survivalists is that the NDE occurs during a period of unconsciousness when the brain has effectively ceased functioning. However, testing this assumption is less straightforward than many might think, as there are some quite major technical and ethical challenges to overcome. Most likely this research would have to be performed in a medical environment. Such a model does actually exist in the form of prospective clinical designs using cardiac arrest patients, about which we go into more detail later on. But confirming brain function in many medical settings, particularly emergency situations, may be complicated to achieve owing to the swift nature of any given crisis event.

Measurement of brain activity by electroencephalogram (EEG) would require that the EEG be attached to the patient already (highly unlikely and not a simple or quick exercise to perform even by experienced operators) and even if such a situation were to occur, the readings from the EEG would be confusing to interpret owing to artefacts induced by the attending staff as they work on the patient (Sartori 2008). Of course, we are talking here about an ideal research situation. In reality, the business of medical staff is to save lives and obtain the best possible outcomes for the people who are entrusted to their care. In that sense, it is doubtful that medical professionals working in operating theatres would be inclined to permit such monitoring. Even if it could be made possible we would still need to establish that the NDE itself actually happened during a period of brain inactivity.

Within the last decade the introduction of the aforementioned prospective clinical study has been a significant addition to the NDE research agenda. Since van Lommel *et al.* (2001) conducted their first prospective study in the Netherlands, several more have been carried out, mostly in the UK (e.g. Parnia *et al.* 2001; Sartori 2008). These kinds of studies have certain distinct methodological advantages. They offer the opportunity to study the NDE in a medical setting, harnessing the skills of a range of health professionals and taking advantage of strict hospital protocols and monitoring equipment. By identifying potential near-death experients as close as possible to the time of their health crisis, interviews and questionnaires can be administered fairly soon in the recovery process, thus overcoming potential memory deficits and distortions – an enduring criticism of studies employing retrospective designs. Yet, much more work needs to be done using this novel approach. Most prospective studies conducted so far have sampled cardiac arrest patients because their cognitive state at the time of their crisis most closely resembles that of the dying brain. However, further work needs to be carried out investigating a range of different illnesses (types and severity) associated with the NDE. So far only one study (van Lommel *et al.* 2001) has utilized a longitudinal research design. There are a plethora of research questions surrounding the long-term health-related aspects of near-death experients. Future prospective studies should be extended to take a broader health-oriented approach, employing a wider range of short- and long-term health measurements, and perhaps also incorporating some form of controlled outcome study of therapeutic approaches to NDE-related problems.

Evidence-based health care is underpinned by rigorous and robust research. The majority of studies carried out in NDE research are nomothetic in nature. These quantitative methodologies have provided us with a wealth of data so far about how the NDE can modify an experient's attitudes and values, but they are ill-equipped to render the fine details of the patient's lived experience of an NDE. In his book *Life After Life* Raymond Moody (1975) observed that no two NDEs are identical. However, the repeated occurrence of certain features in NDE reports from around the world has led some authors to argue for a 'cultural source' theory. Other authors (e.g. Hufford 1982; McClenon 1991, 2010) have disputed this, arguing that NDEs are idiosyncratic and may be based upon the beliefs and expectations of the experient. The importance of the implications of this view cannot be understated. As we have seen in earlier chapters, an experient's reactions to having had an NDE show that time and again radical and life-changing transformations in attitudes, beliefs and lifestyle have occurred. Mostly these changes are experienced positively, but the sudden and intense nature of the NDE can often leave the experient unprepared to cope with any subsequent psycho-social or psycho-spiritual problems. Thus a person can be left fearing for their mental health, confused about how best to communicate their experience to family, friends and health professionals, and, in some cases, with symptoms akin to Post-Traumatic Stress Disorder. All of these can be additional to whatever health issues led them to the point of near-death in the first place. These are very significant health-related issues that deserve sustained research attention.

Several prominent researchers (e.g. Braud 1993; White 1997) have been critical of the lack of research that has been conducted into the significance and impact that NDEs (and other anomalous experiences) have on the people experiencing them. The word 'experience' itself highlights the personal nature of these occurrences. That a near-death *experience* is reported is without question. Whether or not this demonstrates evidence of survival of the human consciousness beyond death is a matter for investigation. From the authors' perspective, an equally important consideration is how a person interprets and draws meaning from that experience, which will partly depend upon if they believe they have survived death or not. As Wilde and Murray (2010, p.58) have recently argued, '…what then may be of great concern to the experient (and researcher) is the "emergence" of the experience into their consciousness. How did the phenomenon initially present itself? What did it feel like?' These considerations cut to the core of what it is to be a person having a lived experience of something out of the ordinary, which is something that has apparently gone missing in the study of NDEs. As Schwartz (1949, p.135) has pointed out, 'in the main [near-death and other anomalous experiences] have been viewed not as human experiences, but as abstract, isolated. That is, the experiences have been studied for their own sake and the human being who had the experience has often been neglected'.

In order to appreciate the experiential components of the NDE from the experient's perspective, researchers need to employ qualitative methods that are sophisticated enough to identify details about the particular nuances of an experient's transformative processes. For example, when a person reports a 'greater interest in spiritual matters' following an NDE, what precisely does that mean or entail for that individual? There remains a need for a deeper exploration of the longitudinal after-effects experienced by people who have NDEs, the nature of those after-effects, and the temporal, social and psychological factors that may impinge on the integration of such an experience, and in particular, the person's sense of self or identity. As Brocki and Wearden (2006) have noted, as modern-day health care experiences a continuing shift from the biomedical model of disease and illness to one that recognizes the constructed nature of illness, health care professionals are sensing the significance of understanding a patient's subjective perceptions and interpretations of their own experiences. Qualitative methods allow both clinician and researcher to comprehend the idiographic nature of the NDE, to explore in depth the dispositional power of the NDE to be a fundamental constituent of an experient's evolving self-identity. It is also important to remember that the meaning and impact of an NDE is not restricted to just the experient, but can radiate out to their family members, friends and peers, as well as other health care professionals with whom they come into contact (see Morris and Knafl 2003).

Data from such methods can vary widely and uniquely, from face-to-face interviews, multi-voiced dialogical accounts taken from online forums and interest groups, focus groups, written testimonies, and experient journals. Furthermore, clinicians may find the active listening skills, reflexivity and sensitivity to context inherent in the presentation of qualitative findings resonant with some of the clinical and communication skills employed in their own everyday practices.

The NDE is a historically recurrent phenomenon, the reports of which have created speculation and controversy amongst lay and professional people alike regarding the true nature of the experience, be that spiritual, psychological or organic (Roe 2001). The search for definitive answers has driven an increasing research interest in all three of these areas. Overall, these endeavours have largely been hampered by a deficiency in the research community in general to precisely define the phenomenon, and a concurrent inability by pro-survivalists in particular to produce theories of the NDE that generate falsifiable hypotheses. By contrast, neuroscientific research has stolen quite a march in this respect, but it has yet to provide a comprehensive, empirically supported account of the NDE. However, research into the area of personal meaning and transformation is one that the authors believe may be particularly fertile and which can be conducted largely independent of the issue of veridicality. By examining the experience and meaning that experients apportion to their NDEs, such research findings can better furnish psychologists and health care professionals to understand their clients' experiences and to help them with any potential personality transformations or psycho-spiritual crises that may arise in response to these most fascinating of life events.

Conclusion

This book has been written with the focus on improving health professionals' understanding of near-death experiences (NDEs) so that they could assess this phenomenon more efficiently and provide necessary support and guidance for those who have experienced it. When a reader goes through different chapters, it might be challenging to remember essential information in all the chapters of the book. To make it easy for the readers, this chapter will recapitulate key information.

To begin with, what is worth remembering is that accounts of NDEs have been in existence since time immemorial. Systematic investigation of this phenomenon has clearly substantiated the occurrence of this phenomenon in both life-threatening and non life-threatening situations. Following combined efforts of scientists with great interest in this field, an international organization – International Organization for Near-Death Studies (IANDS) – has been formed. Further, NDE has been defined to include both the nature of the experience and the circumstances of its occurrence.

Critical evaluation of available studies indicate limitations in some of these studies but what is important to note is that there is a relative consensus that NDE occurs in a small proportion of the general population, 4–9 per cent. Nonetheless, studies including high-risk population (participants who have faced life-threatening situations) report an average of 25 per cent, with no NDEs in some studies and almost all having the experience in others.

Certain features of NDE are noted commonly and it is not necessary that an individual needs to have all the experiences. Broadly speaking,

NDEs could be pleasant (in the majority) or unpleasant. In general, a high proportion of individuals with this experience go through positive transformation in their life. A striking feature is the universality of consciousness as evidenced in some of the narratives and the feelings of love, the ephemeral nature and transcendence. It by no means takes away the fear component faced by others. Since these experiences do generally have a profound impact on the individual and also may create secondary problems to those around him/her we need to be in a position to understand and help the aforesaid if and when the need arises.

There are instruments to measure this phenomenon with a considerable degree of objectivity. Their application in the studies is recommended. Careful review and planning of study methodology will assist in future research work and in meta-analytic studies.

There are unique aspects in childhood NDEs, for example, being accompanied into the light. On the other hand, as in adult experiences, child experiences are generally pleasant and positively transforming.

There are a number of theoretical explanations for NDEs. Recently, there is an increased interest in neurobiological propositions. Particularly, a neural substance – DMT – and pineal gland are gaining greater attention. Given the complexity of these experiences and the limitations of such theories, it is reasonable to state that aetiological explanations remain inconclusive.

Although the occurrence of NDEs has no relation to demographic variables, particularly age and sex, the expression and the interpretation of such experiences vary to a degree in different cultures. Clinicians need to be cognizant of such cultural variations to effectively identify and help the experiencer. The description of an NDE by an individual is obviously influenced but not limited to his/her linguistic capabilities. Other factors that are likely to have a bearing are social, religious and other idiosyncratic features.

While assessing individuals who report NDEs, health care professionals need to assess associated conditions such as consequences of brain injury and psychological consequences. Further, the psychopathological states, medical conditions and other spiritual experiences that look like NDEs need to be differentiated.

End-of-life experiences occur in individuals faced with terminal illnesses. These experiences are akin to NDEs and it will be highly relevant for clinicians in palliative care to equip themselves with knowledge of these experiences to improve the quality of care.

Management strategies involve support and encouragement to talk about individuals' experiences. With support, over a period of time, individuals tend to integrate these experiences. Although negative after-effects are less often reported, clinicians need to be aware of this possibility so that screening could be done for such negative states. Psychological interventions in the form of support, validation, empathy and guidance, and social approaches in the form of sharing personal experiences in a group setting (connecting with individuals who have had similar experiences) and connecting with a larger group via web resources such as www.iands.org or www.nde.net.au are generally helpful.

Future research in NDEs will need to focus on its veridical nature, obtaining more precise epidemiological data and the long-term effects of this experience and comparing the lives of the NDErs with matched controls.

Interview Schedule

Date(s) of interview:

Name of interviewer:

Name of interviewee:

Condition of the patient at time of interview:

Circumstances of the interview (other persons, noise, interruptions, and so forth):

(In introducing yourself to the patient, you should explain the purpose of the interview pretty much as follows. These initial comments should be as standardized as possible across interviewers and hospitals.)

Hello, my name is_____. I'm a [*graduate student, professor*] at_____. How are you feeling today? *(Take whatever time necessary to establish rapport with patient.)* I believe_____ [*name of contact*] told you a little about why I wanted to speak with you. Some associates and I at the University of _____are working on a project concerned with what people experience when they undergo a life-threatening situation, like having a serious illness or accident. I understand that you recently may have experienced such an occurrence. Is that right? *(Wait for patient to respond.)* Naturally it is extremely helpful to us to be able to speak with people who have had this kind of experience themselves; that's why I'm grateful to you for being willing to talk to me about this. So, in a few minutes I'd like to ask you some questions that I've prepared for this purpose, but first let me mention a few things that may help us.

The first thing I should say is that some people – not necessarily everyone, though – appear to experience some unusual things when they have a serious illness or accident or when they come close to dying. Sometimes these things are a little puzzling and people are somewhat hesitant to talk about them. *(Be a little jocular here; try by your manner to put the patient at ease.)* Now please don't worry about this in talking with me! I just want you to feel free to tell me anything

---

*   Reproduced with permission from the author. These questionnaires appeared in Ring, K. (1980) *Life at Death: A Scientific Investigation of Near-Death Experience.* New York: Coward, McCann and Geoghegan.

you can remember – whether it makes sense to you or not, OK? *(Wait for patient to respond.)*

Now let me assure you about one further thing. These interviews will be held in strictest confidence. When we analyse our results, any information you may furnish us will never be identified by name. Since we can guarantee that these interviews will be kept anonymous and confidential, you can feel free to tell me whatever you wish without having to worry that others may learn of your private experience.

As you may remember from the informed consent sheet you signed, Mr [Mrs, Ms]_____, we are going to tape-record this interview. This is standard practice in these studies and makes it possible to have an absolutely accurate record of what you say without my having to try to write everything down. Naturally, the tape-recorded material will also be available *only* to my associates.

We hope we'll be able to complete this interview today, but it you should grow tired, please let me know and we shall complete it another time. After we're finished, I would be happy to answer any [further] questions you may have, but I think it would be best if I spoke with you first.

(Turn tape cassette on at this point – and make sure to check it for sound level; an inaudible or poorly audible recording is useless to us.)

(Interview proper begins here.)

Now, Mr [Mrs, Ms]_____. I first need to ask you just a few questions about yourself. First of all, may I know your *age*, please? What is your *occupation*? What is the *highest grade* you completed in school? May I know your *religious preference* or affiliation, please, if you have one. *(Also make note of race, sex; if apparently foreign, get nationality. All this should be written down on the prepared form even though it is on tape.)* Are you *married*? *(If not, find out what marital status is: Widowed? Divorced? Single? Separated?)*

Now, according to _____ [*name of contact*], you recently _____*[specify condition, for example, attempted suicide, had a serious accident, illness, experienced cardiac arrest, and so forth]*. Can you tell me how this came about? *(Let patient narrate this as much as possible in his/her own words, but probe, as necessary, for pertinent details if not otherwise forthcoming: date, location, circumstances, witnesses, and so on. Try to get patient to describe circumstances as specifically as possible.)*

Sometimes people report experiencing certain things during an incident like yours. Do you remember being aware of anything while you _____ *[specify condition]*. Could you describe this for me? *(Probe here, if necessary, for any feelings, perceptions, imagery, visions, and so forth. Try to make the patient aware that you understand that some aspects of his/her experience may be difficult or impossible to put into words. If you think it would facilitate matters, give patient a paper and pencil in case he/*

she would prefer to depict some aspect of his/her experience visually. But again, allow the patient to describe the experience in his/her own words as much as possible.)

Now, I'd like to ask you certain more specific questions about your experience. *(For those patients who report no awareness during their episode, say, 'Even though you don't recall anything specific from this time, let me just ask you whether any of these things rings a bell with you.)*

(Modify this section, as necessary, depending on what a patient has previously said.)

1. Was the kind of experience difficult to put into words? *(If yes:)* Can you try all the same to tell me why? What was it about the experience that makes it so hard to communicate? Was it like a dream or different from a dream? *(Probe.)*

2. When this episode occurred, *did you think you were dying or close to death? Did you actually think you were dead? (Important questions to ask!)* Did you hear anyone actually say that you were dead? What else do you recall hearing while in this state? *(Ask these questions in turn.)*

3. What were your feelings and sensations during the episode?

4. Did you hear any noises or unusual sounds during the episode?

5. Did you at any time feel as though you were travelling or moving? What was that experience like? *(If appropriate:)* Was this experience in any way associated with the noise (or sound) you described before?

6. Did you at any time during this experience feel that you were somehow separate from your own physical body? During this time, were you ever aware of *seeing* your physical body? *(Ask these questions in turn. Then, if appropriate, ask:)* Could you describe this experience for me? How did you feel when you were in this state? Do you recall any thoughts that you had when you were in this state? When you were outside your own physical body, where were you? Did you have another body? *(If yes:)* Was there any kind of connection between yourself and your physical body? Any kind of link between the two that you could see? Describe it for me. When you were in this state, what were your perceptions of time? Of space? Of weight? Is there anything you could do while in this state that you could not do in your ordinary physical body? Were you aware of any tastes or odours? How, if at all, were your vision and hearing affected while in this state? Did you experience a sense of loneliness while in this state? How so? *(Ask these questions in turn.)*

7. During your episode, did you ever encounter other individuals, living or dead? *(If affirmative:)* Who were they? What happened when you met them? Did they communicate to you? What? How? Why do you think they communicated what they did to you? How did you feel in their presence?

8. Did you at any time experience a light, glow, or illumination? Can you describe this to me? *(If affirmative:)* Did this 'light' communicate anything to you? What? What did you make of this light? How did you feel? *(Or how did it make you feel?)* Did you encounter any religious figures such as angels, guardian spirits, Christ, and so forth? Did you encounter any frightening spirits such as demons, witches, or the devil? *(Ask questions in turn.)*

9. When you were going through this experience, did your life – or scenes from your life – ever appear to you as mental images or memories? *(If so:)* Can you describe this to me further? What was this experience like? How did it make you feel? Did you feel you learned anything from this experience? If so, what? *(Ask questions in turn.)*

10. Did you at any time have a sense of approaching some kind of boundary or limit or threshold or point of no return? *(If so:)* Can you describe this to me? Did you have any particular feelings or thoughts that you can recall as you approached this boundary? *(Ask questions in turn.)* Do you have any idea what this boundary represented or meant?

11. *(If patient has previously stated that he/she came close to dying, ask:)* When you felt close to dying, how did you feel? Did you want to come back to your body, to life? How did it feel when you did find yourself conscious again in your own body? Do you have any recollection of how you got back into your physical body? Do you have any idea why you didn't die at this time? Did you ever feel judged by some impersonal force? *(Ask questions in turn.)*

12. This experience of yours has been (very) recent but I wonder if you feel it has changed you in any way. Do you think so or not? If it has changed you, in what way? *(If necessary and appropriate, then ask:)* Has this experience changed your attitude toward life? How? Has it altered your religious beliefs? If so, how? Compared to how you felt before this experience, are you more or less afraid of death, or the same? *(If appropriate:)* Are you afraid of death at all? *(If patient had attempted suicide, ask:)* How has this experience affected your attitude toward suicide? How likely is it that you might try to commit suicide again? *(Be tactful.)* *(Ask these questions in turn.)*

13. *(If this has not been fully covered in Question 12, then ask, if patient has stated that he/she has come close to dying:)* As one who has come close to dying, can you tell me, in your own way, what you now understand death to be? What does death now mean to you?

14. Is there anything else you'd like to add here concerning this experience or its effects on you?

Religious beliefs and practices

Now, I have just a few more brief questions to ask you and then we'll be done. This time I'd like you to answer these questions from two points of view: how things were *before* this incident occurred and how things were *afterward*. Do you understand? *(Make sure patient does.)* If you feel that something *remained the same afterward* as it had been before, just say 'same', OK? *(Record responses on the appropriate form.)*

1. Before this incident occurred, how religious a person would you say you were: very religious? Quite religious? Fairly religious? Not too religious? Not religious at all? *(If patient selects last alternative, ask him/her if he/she would call him/herself an atheist or non-believer.)* How would you classify yourself now? *(If patient has previously classified him/herself as a non-believer, ask him/her if this has remained the same.)*

2. Before, how strongly would you say you believed in God: absolute belief in God? Strong belief? Fairly strong belief? Not too strong belief? No belief at all? How about now?

3. Before, how convinced were you that there was such a thing as life after death: completely convinced? Strongly convinced? Tended to believe there was? Not sure? Tended to doubt it? Didn't believe it at all? How about now?

4. Before, did you believe in heaven? In hell? How about now? *(If patient's views have changed, encourage him/her to say why. We are especially interested in his/her conception of hell here, so try to solicit his/her views on that especially.)*

5. Before, had you read, thought or heard about the kind of experience you came to have? Do you recall seeing anything about this sort of thing on TV, in books and magazines, and so forth? *(Try to find out specifically what patient has seen or read.) (If appropriate:)* Have you had time or the inclination to look into this matter since your own experience? Have you talked with anyone besides me about the experience? Who? When was this? Do you remember what you talked about? *(Ask these questions in turn.)*

(This ends the formal portion of the interview.)

Well, Mr [Mrs, Ms]_____, that's all the questions I have. Do you have any you'd like to ask me? *(Answer these questions in however much detail the patient seems interested to hear no matter how long it takes—even if you have to make an extra trip back to do so; consider it part of your job.)*

(When this is done) Mr [Mrs, Ms] _____, I want to thank you very much for your willingness to grant us this interview. Your comments will be of great help to us in our research and if you're interested, we'd be happy to send you a brief report of our findings when our research is completed. Would

you be interested in this? *(If patient expresses interest, obtain an address where the report can be sent.)*

Now, if for any reason, Mr [Mrs, Ms]_____, you should wish to get in touch with me, this is my name and phone number – or you can write to me at this address. *(Give either home address or university address. Have cards typed or printed up for distribution.)*

I'll gather my things together now. Thank you again for helping us out. *(If it applies:)* We'll send you a copy of our report when our preliminary work is finished. *(If appropriate, wish the patient a speedy recovery or good health – or at least diminished pain. Don't leave, however, until you've done all you can, if necessary, to relieve any stress or anxiety the interview may have occasioned.)*

Tape Rating Form

Respondent: _____ Rater: _____

Coding symbols and instructions

Use + + if a characteristic is present *and* strong, vivid, stressed, or otherwise compelling.

Use + if a characteristic is present.

Use ? if a characteristic might have been present.

Use – if a characteristic has been inquired about *and* is either denied or not present.

Make no mark next to a characteristic that is not mentioned.

In the space for comments, write down any memorable quotes verbatim or indicate that there is good, quotable material by writing a large Q in the relevant space. Also use this space to note anything pertinent to your ratings or to the comments of the respondent.

With regard to uncertainty concerning the proper section to note *feelings* or *sensations*, when in doubt make your entries in Section D, along with any appropriate comments.

---

* Reproduced with permission from the author. These questionnaires appeared in Ring, K. (1980) *Life at Death: A Scientific Investigation of the Near-Death Experience.* New York: Coward, McCann and Geoghegan.

Characteristics	Rating	Comments
A. Ineffability of experience		
B. Subjective sense of dying		
C. Subjective sense of being dead		
D. Feeling and sensations at time of near-death experience (use 22–25 at the end of this list to specify others)		
1. Peacefulness		
2. Calmness		
3. Quiet		
4. Serenity		
5. Lightness		
6. Warmth		
7. Pleasantness		
8. Happiness		
9. Joy, exaltation		
10. Painlessness		
11. Relief		
12. No fear		
13. Relaxation		
14. Resignation		
15. Curiosity		
16. Anxiety		
17. Fear		
18. Anger		
19. Dread		
20. Despair		
21. Anguish		
22.		
23.		
24.		
25.		
E. Unusual noise(s); if +, describe		

Characteristics	Rating	Comments
F. Sense of movement, location		
1. Quality of movement, experience		
a. Walking		
b. Running		
c. Floating		
d. Flying		
e. Movement without body		
f. Dreamlike		
g. Echoic		
h.		
i.		
2. Feelings on moving		
a. Peaceful		
b. Exhilarating		
c. Struggling		
d. Fearful		
e. Panicky		
f.		
g.		
3. Sensed features of location		
a. Dark void		
b. Tunnel		
c. Path, road		
d. Garden		
e. Valley		
f. Meadow		
g. Fields		
h. City		
i. Illumination of scene		
j. Vivid colours		
k. Music		
l. Human figures		
m. Other beings		
n.		
o.		
p.		

Characteristics		Rating	Comments
G.	Sense of bodily separation		
	1. Felt detached from body, but did not see it		
	2. Able to view body		
	3. Sense of time		
	a. Undistorted		
	b. No sense of time		
	c. Timelessness		
	d.		
	4. Sense of space		
	a. Undistorted		
	b. No sense of space		
	c. Infinite, no boundaries		
	d.		
	5. Feeling bodily weight		
	a. Ordinary bodily weight		
	b. Light		
	c. Weightlessness		
	d. No sense of body		
	e.		
	6. Sense of loneliness		
H.	Presence of others		
	1. Deceased relative(s); if +, specify		
	2. Deceased friend		
	3. Guide, voice		
	4. Jesus		
	5. God, the Lord, a higher power, etc.		
	6. Angels		
	7. Evil spirits, devil, etc.		
	8. Living person(s); if +, specify		
I.	Light, illumination		
	1. Colour(s)		
	2. Hurt eyes?		

Characteristics		Rating	Comments
J.	Life flashbacks		
	1. Complete		
	2. Highpoints		
	3. Other (specify)		
	4. Sense of sequence		
K.	Threshold effect		
L.	Feelings upon recovery		
	1. Not relevant		
	2. Anger		
	3. Resentment		
	4. Disappointment		
	5. Shock		
	6. Pain		
	7. Relief		
	8. Peace		
	9. Happiness		
	10. Gladness		
	11. Joy		
	12.		

Characteristics	Rating	Comments
M. Changes		
1. Attitude toward life		
a. Increased appreciation		
b. More caring, loving		
c. Renewed sense of purpose		
d. Fear, feeling of vulnerability		
e. More interested, curious		
f.		
2. Religious beliefs/attitudes		
a. Stronger		
b. Weaker		
c. Other (specify)		
3. Fear of death		
a. Greater		
b. Lesser		
c. None		
N. Idea of death		
1. Annihilation		
2. Body dies, soul survives		
3. Transitional state		
4. Continuance of life at another level		
5. Merging with universal consciousness		
6. Reincarnation ideas		
7. Peace		
8. Bliss		
9. A beautiful experience		
10. A journey		
11. No idea		
12. Nothing, nothingness		
13.		
14.		

Near-Death Experience Scale

Please circle one number (0, 1 or 2) for each question to indicate which answer comes closest to what you experienced during your NDE:

1. Did time seem to speed up or slow down?

    0 = No

    1 = Time seemed to go faster or slower than usual

    2 = Everything seemed to be happening at once; or time stopped or lost all meaning

2. Were your thoughts speeded up?

    0 = No

    1 = Faster than usual

    2 = Incredibly fast

3. Did scenes from your past come back to you?

    0 = No

    1 = I remembered many past events

    2 = My past flashed before me, out of my control

4. Did you suddenly seem to understand everything?

    0 = No

    1 = Everything about myself or others

    2 = Everything about the universe

5. Did you have a feeling of peace or pleasantness?

    0 = No

    1 = Relief or calmness

    2 = Incredible peace or pleasantness

---

*   Reproduced with permission from Professor Bruce Greyson

6. Did you have a feeling of joy?

    0 = No

    1 = Happiness

    2 = Incredible joy

7. Did you feel a sense of harmony or unity with the universe?

    0 = No

    1 = I felt no longer in conflict with nature

    2 = I felt united or one with the world

8. Did you see, or feel surrounded by, a brilliant light?

    0 = No

    1 = An unusually bright light

    2 = A light clearly of mystical or other-worldly origin

9. Were your senses more vivid than usual?

    0 = No

    1 = More vivid than usual

    2 = Incredibly more vivid

10. Did you seem to be aware of things going on elsewhere, as if by extrasensory perception (ESP)?

    0 = No

    1 = Yes, but the facts have not been checked out

    2 = Yes, and the facts have been checked out

11. Did scenes from the future come to you?

    0 = No

    1 = Scenes from my personal future

    2 = Scenes from the world's future

12. Did you feel separated from your body?

    0 = No

    1 = I lost awareness of my body

    2 = I clearly left my body and existed outside it

13. Did you seem to enter some other, unearthly world?

    0 = No

    1 = Some unfamiliar and strange place

    2 = A clearly mystical or unearthly realm

14. Did you seem to encounter a mystical being or presence, or hear an unidentifiable voice?

   0 = No

   1 = I heard a voice I could not identify

   2 = I encountered a definite being, or a voice clearly of mystical or unearthly origin

15. Did you see deceased or religious spirits?

   0 = No

   1 = I sensed their presence

   2 = I actually saw them

16. Did you come to a border or point of no return?

   0 = No

   1 = I came to a definite conscious decision to 'return' to life

   2 = I came to a barrier that I was not permitted to cross; or was 'sent back' against my will

The NDE Scale score is the sum of the ratings for all 16 items. Possible scores therefore range from 0 to 32. The mean score among a large sample of near-death experiencers is 15, with a standard deviation of 8. We have designated a minimum score of 7 (one standard deviation below the mean) as the criterion for identifying an experience as an NDE.

   Within the NDE Scale, there are four components that reflect different aspects of the NDE and can be scored separately. Each of these components thus has possible scores ranging from 0 to 8. Items 1 to 4 constitute the Cognitive Component, reflecting changes in thought processes. Items 5 to 8 constitute the Affective Component, reflecting changes in emotional state. Items 9 to 12 constitute the Paranormal Component, reflecting purported paranormal phenomena in the mundane realm. Items 13 to 16 constitute the Transcendental Component, reflecting apparent experiences of an extramundane dimension or realm of existence.

NDE Questionnaire

NDQ 1. At any time in your life have you ever felt that you were close to the point of dying?

- Yes

- No

- Can't say

If ever been close to dying, ask:
NDQ 2. Can you briefly describe the situation that you were in when this happened? *If necessary prompt:* What situations were you in when you had this near-death experience?

- Cardiac arrest/heart attack

- Motor accident

- Suicide attempt

- Critical illness

- Coma

- Nearly drowned

- Combat situation

- Childbirth complications

- Psychological illness/condition

- During/after medical operation

- Doing stupid things (unspecified)

- Drug overdose

- Other medical condition/illness

- Adverse reaction to medication

---

* Reproduced with permission from the principal author, Dr Mahendra Perera and the Editor-in-chief, Janice Holden *Journal of Near-Death Studies*. The questionnaire appeared in Perera, M., Padmasekara, G. and Belanti, J. (2005) 'Prevalence of near-death experiences in Australia.' *Journal of Near-Death Studies 24*, 109–116.

- Was shot at (non-combat)
- Domestic squabble
- Electric shock
- Other (specify)
- Can't say

NDQ_3. What, if anything, did you see or hear or feel during this near-death experience? What else? Anything else? *(no prompt is used)*

- Out-of-body experience/felt as though outside my body
- Saw a light
- Saw a tunnel
- Saw deceased spirits/people who had died
- Saw religious figures/Gods/angels
- Felt I was going to heaven/hell/purgatory/other unearthly place
- Had a feeling of peace
- Heard noises (pleasant/unpleasant)
- Other (specify)
- Can't say
- Nothing

NDQ_4. In that near-death situation did any of the following things happen? *(Prompt by reading out and highlight all mentioned.)*

- Out-of-body experience
- Seeing light, tunnel
- Spirits of deceased persons
- Gods, angels, or other religious figures
- Feeling in unearthly places – heaven or hell, peace, pleasant or unpleasant noises
- None of the above

The Contributors

P.M.H. Atwater LHD is one of the original researchers in the field of near-death studies, having begun her work in 1978 and written ten books on her findings. Her summary work is *Near-Death Experiences: The Rest of The Story*. In 2005, IANDS presented her with an Outstanding Service Award, and the National Association of Transpersonal Hypnotherapists awarded her a Lifetime Achievement Award. In 2010, she was also awarded the Nancy E. Bush Award for Literary Excellence and the Lifetime Achievement and Special Services Award, both from IANDS. Dr Atwater is a noted authority on NDE after-effects, children's cases, and hellish NDEs. She has experienced three NDEs herself, and has had sessions with nearly 4000 adult and child experiencers. In 2001, her work on NDE after-effects was cited in *The Lancet*.

Paul Badham PhD is Emeritus Professor of Theology and Religious Studies at University of Wales Trinity Saint David. He is a graduate in Theology from the Universities of Oxford and Cambridge and was supervised for his PhD by John Hick at the University of Birmingham. Since 1973 he has taught Theology and Religious Studies in the University of Wales where he has been a professor since 1992. From 2002 to 2010 he was Director of the Alister Hardy Religious Experience Research Centre. He directed an MA in Death and Immortality for over 20 years. His publications include *Christian Beliefs about Life after Death* (1976), *Immortality or Extinction?* (1982), *Death and Immortality in the Religions of the World* (1987), *Ethics on the Frontiers of Human Existence* (1992), *Facing Death* (1996), and *Is there a Christian Case for Assisted Dying?* (2010).

John Belanti BSW, MAASW (Acc) is a Social Worker and Team Leader in North West Continuing Care Team, North West Area Mental Health Service, Melbourne, Australia. Over the past eight years, he has engaged in research in the Prevalence of Near-Death Experiences in Australia and explored Cross-Cultural Phenomenology of Near-Death Experiences. In the clinical field, he supervises and supports clinicians, clients and carers in working through issues particularly relating to mental health, grief, loss and mindfulness. In 2004, he was a witness and survivor of a major tsunami and used these experiences to inform his professional development and clinical practice. John continues to promote awareness of near-death experience (NDE) to clinicians and students in the adult mental health field. He has interest in healing therapies such as meditation, clinical hypnosis and Reiki.

Ornella Corazza MA, PhD is a medical anthropologist who specializes in substance misuse, medical law/ethics and intercultural communication. She works as Research Manager for the Recreational Drugs European Network (ReDNet) a Europe-wide research project on public health funded by the European Commission at the School of Pharmacy, University of Hertfordshire and King's College, Institute of Psychiatry, in London. She has held fellowships at the University of Padua (Italy), University of Bochum (Germany) and University of Tokyo (Japan), where she has studied the NDEs among the Japanese. She is author of various academic publications, including the recent book *Near-Death Experiences: Exploring the Mind–Body Connection* (Routledge, 2008).

Peter Fenwick MB, BChir, DPM, FRCPsych is Consultant Neuropsychiatrist Emeritus to the Epilepsy Unit at the Maudsley Hospital which he ran for 20 years. His current appointments include: Senior Lecturer at the Institute of Psychiatry, Consultant Neuropsychiatrist at the Radcliffe Infirmary Oxford and Honorary Consultant Clinical Neurophysiologist at Broadmoor Hospital. He is a past Chairman of the Scientific and Medical Network and is Chairman of the Research Committee for the Foundation for Integrated Medicine. He has had a long-standing interest in brain function, the relationship of the mind and the brain, and the problem of consciousness. He has an extensive research record and has published over 200 papers in medical and scientific journals on brain function and also several papers on meditation and altered states of consciousness. He is widely regarded as the main clinical authority in the UK on the subject of NDEs and is highly regarded by both medical colleagues and the media for his knowledge of this subject.

Karuppiah Jagadheesan, MBBS, MD, FRANZCP is a consultant psychiatrist working in general adult psychiatry. He is currently working at North West Continuing Care Team and Community Care Units, North West Area Mental Health Service, Melbourne, Australia. He has a keen interest in the investigation of psychopathological states and has published several articles in well-known journals. Along with Dr Mahendra Perera and John Belanti, he has been involved in exploring NDEs in individuals with mental health needs and supporting them to deal with these experiences whilst promoting awareness among mental health professionals.

Rohan Jayasuriya MBBS, MD, MPH is a researcher in Behavioural Medicine and an epidemiologist. He has an interest in methods used to study psychosomatic disease and chronic illness. He has taught epidemiology and critical appraisal methods at the University of Wollongong and University of New South Wales, Australia. In his current research, he uses cognitive behavioural interventions for management of chronic disease.

Lalith Kuruppuarachchi MBBS, MD, FRPsych (UK) graduated from the University of Peradeniya, Sri Lanka with his basic medical degree in 1982. He has completed his postgraduate psychiatric training in Sri Lanka and was awarded an MD in Psychiatry by the Post Graduate Institute of Medicine, University of Colombo, Sri Lanka in 1988. He was further trained in psychiatry in the Newcastle Rotational Training Scheme, UK and obtained a MRCPsych (UK) in spring 1992. He was elected to the Fellowship of the Royal College of Psychiatrists, UK in February 2006. He was the founder head of the Department of Psychiatry, Faculty of Medicine, University of Kelaniya, Ragama, Sri Lanka and appointed to the Chair in Psychiatry in 2004 and has been the Professor of Psychiatry, University of Kelaniya, Sri Lanka since 2004.

He is actively involved in undergraduate and postgraduate psychiatric education/training and is currently a member of the Board of Study in Psychiatry, Post-Graduate Institute of Medicine, University of Colombo, Sri Lanka. He has widely published his work in National and International peer-reviewed journals, contributed to several book chapters related to psychiatry and published a book in native language related to mental health. He recently developed an interest in NDE and engaged in studies in NDE with his colleagues.

Craig Murray, PhD, PGCE is an academic based at Lancaster University. He carries out qualitative research into chronic illness and mental health with a particular emphasis on implications for clinical psychologists and services. This has most recently involved examining caregivers' experiences of caring for a husband with Parkinson's disease and psychotic symptoms, an analysis of delusions in people with Parkinson's disease, and co-constructions of couplehood by couples when one partner has dementia. Other current research projects include recovery from bipolar disorder (with the Spectrum Centre), the experience of CBT for PTSD, and suicide prevention (with Manchester University). Other clinical topics in which he is research active include self-harm, anomalous experiences, and mental health following amputation. In 2009 he was editor of a book entitled *Psychological Scientific Perspectives on Out-of-Body and Near-Death Experiences* (Nova Science Publishers, New York).

Satwant Pasricha PhD is the former Professor and Head (Chair), Department of Clinical Psychology, National Institute of Mental Health and Neuroscience, (NIMHANS), Bangalore, India where she was engaged in teaching, patient care and research. She joined NIMHANS as a faculty member in December 1980 as a lecturer in clinical parapsychology, became full professor of clinical psychology in 2000 and worked there till February 2009. Her research interest has been in the survival of human personality beyond death and mind–brain relationship. She is the only person in India carrying out systematic investigations into cases of the reincarnation type, NDEs and other paranormal experiences (mostly in collaboration with the late Professor Ian Stevenson of the University of Virginia) since 1974. She became a post-doctoral fellow at the Department of Psychiatry and Behavioral Medicine, School of Medicine, University of Virginia, USA in 1979 and has subsequently visited there several times in different capacities. She has published nearly 50 articles in reputed scientific journals and has authored two books, *Claims of Reincarnation: An Empirical Study of Cases in India* (Harman Publishing House, 1989/2006) and *Can the Mind Survive beyond Death? In Pursuit of Scientific Evidence* (two volumes) (Harman Publishing House, 2008). Currently Dr Pasricha has settled in Dehra Dun and is engaged full time in research on paranormal experiences and is also working on a book on NDEs.

Anthony Peake is a graduate of the University of Warwick and a postgraduate of the London School of Economics. Anthony's previous books and articles present a concept that he terms 'cheating the ferryman' (CTF). This concept, a totally original theory about what happens to human consciousness at the point of death was first presented in an academic paper published in the *Journal of Near-Death Studies* in 2004. Such was the power of this idea that the editor of the periodical, Dr Bruce Greyson, Carlson Professor of Psychiatry at the University of Virginia, was subsequently to describe it as 'the most innovative and provocative argument that I have ever seen'. Anthony is a member of the Scientific & Medical Network (SMN), The Society For Psychical Research (SPR), The Institute of Noetic Sciences (IONS) and a professional member of the International Association of Near-Death Studies. Anthony is one of a selection of individuals who will be featured in a forthcoming book entitled *Visionaries for the 21st Century*. Anthony's 'vision statement' will appear with statements from such luminaries as Jonathon Porrit, James O'Dea, William Tiller, Neale Donald Walsch, Alice Walker and Jane Goodall.

Mahendra Perera graduated from the University of Ceylon Peradeniya with his basic medical degree. A doctoral thesis on benzodiazepine dependence was completed at the University of Sheffield, and he has obtained postgraduate qualifications in psychiatry in Sri Lanka (MD), Australia (FRANZCP) and the UK (MRCPsych). Mahendra is also a foundation Fellow of the Chapter of Addiction Medicine, in the Royal Australasian College of Physicians. Mahendra is currently engaged in private practice in Melbourne as a consultant psychiatrist and an Honorary Senior Fellow of the University of Melbourne.

Mahendra is on the General Medical Council (UK) specialist register as well as registered with the Sri Lankan Medical Council in addition to the licence to practise in Australia. As a fellow of the Melbourne University he is engaged in teaching medical students as well as teaching psychiatry trainees. He is currently involved in a research project in Sri Lanka studying the prevalence of NDEs in a General Hospital population.

Mahendra has published work in peer-reviewed journals regularly and the most recent work has been in the field of NDEs and culture-related illness.

Cherie Sutherland PhD is the author of five books on NDEs and related subjects. She is a sociologist, educator and researcher. For over 15 years she has been a shamanic practitioner and maintained a private counselling practice in Byron Bay, Australia. She also runs shamanic workshops and lectures widely throughout Australia on the subject of NDEs, after-death visits, shamanism and angels.

Pim van Lommel MD was a world-renowned cardiologist. Since his initial study of NDEs, which was published in the prestigious medical journal *The Lancet*, Dr van Lommel has resigned his post as a practising cardiologist to devote his time to further research and lecturing all over the world on NDEs. He is the author of *Consciousness Beyond Life: The Science of the Near-Death Experience*.

David Wilde BSc gained his undergraduate BSc in Psychology with Human Physiology at the University of Sunderland in 1996. Following that he graduated with an MSc in Environmental Psychology at the University of Surrey in 1997. He spent the next seven years working as a research associate in the fields of environmental psychology and palliative care. In 2005, David attained a Diploma in Consciousness and Transpersonal Psychology from Liverpool John Moore's University. In the same year he joined the School of Psychological Sciences at the University of Manchester, where he began working on his PhD investigating the occurrence and phenomenology of out-of-body and NDEs. Currently David is working at the University of Huddersfield on a Macmillan Cancer Support funded project and writing up his PhD, which he hopes to submit in July 2011.

References

Foreword

Foster, R., James, D. and Holden, J.M. (2009). 'Practical Applications of Research on Near-Death Experiences.' In J. M. Holden, B. Greyson and D. James (eds.), *The Handbook of Near-Death Experiences: Thirty Years of Investigation* (pp. 235–258). Santa Barbara, CA: Praeger/ABC-CLIO.

Holden, J.M., Greyson, B. and James, D. (2009). 'The Field of Near-Death Studies: Past, Present, and Future.' In J. M. Holden, B. Greyson, and D. James (eds.), *The Handbook of Near-Death Experiences: Thirty Years of Investigation* (pp. 1–16). Santa Barbara, CA: Praeger/ABC-CLIO.

Holden, J.M., Oden, K., Kozlowski, K. and Hayslip, B. (2011). Teaching about near-death experiences: The effectiveness of using *The Day I Died*. *Omega – The Journal of Death and Dying, 63*, 4, 373–388.

Zingrone, N.L. and Alvarado, C.S. (2009). 'Pleasurable Western adult near-death experiences: Features, circumstances, and incidence.' In J. M. Holden, B. Greyson and D. James (eds.), *The Handbook of Near-Death Experiences: Thirty Years of Investigation* (pp. 17–40). Santa Barbara, CA: Praeger/ABC-CLIO.

Chapter 1

Atwater, P.M.H. (1980) *I Died Three Times in 1977*. Dayton, VA. (Self-published).

Atwater, P.M.H. and Morgan, D.H. (2000) *The Complete Idiot's Guide to Near-Death Experiences*. Indianapolis, IN: Alpha Books.

Atwater, P.M.H. (2007) *The Big Book of Near-Death Experiences*. Charlottesville, VA: Hampton Roads.

Gallup, G. and Proctor, W. (1982) *Adventures in Immortality*. New York, NY: McGraw Hill.

Greyson, B. and Flynn, C. (1984) *The Near-Death Experience: Problems, Prospects, Perspectives*. Springfield, IL: C.C. Thomas.

Holden, J. Personal communication

Kelly, E.W., Greyson, B., Kelly, E.F. (2007) 'Unusual Experiences Near-death and Related Phenomena.' In E.F. Kelly, E.W. Kelly, A. Crabtree, A. Gauld, M. Grosso, B. Greyson (eds) *Irreducible Mind: Toward a Psychology for the 21st Century*. Lanham, MD: Rowman and Littlefield.

Kübler-Ross, E. (1991) *On Life after Death*. Berkeley and Toronto: Celestial Arts.

Moody, R.A. (1975) *Life After Life*. Covington, GA: Mockingbird Books.

Ring, K. (1980) *Life at Death*. New York, NY: Coward, McCann and Geoghegan.

Ring, K. (1982) *Life at Death: A Scientific Investigation of Near-Death Experience*. New York, NY: Quill (first published in 1980).

Ring, K. (1984) *Heading Toward Omega: In Search of the Meaning of the Near-Death Experience*. New York City, NY: William Morrow.

Ring, K. and Valarino, E.E. (2006) *Lessons from the Light*. Massachusetts: Moment Point Press (first published in 1998).

Ritchie, G.G. and Sherill, E. (1978) *Return from Tomorrow*. Waco, TX: Chosen Books.

Sheeler, R.D. (2005) 'Teaching near-death experiences to medical students'. *Journal of Near-Death Studies 23*, 239–247.

van Lommel, P. (2005) 'Consciousness and the brain: A new concept about the continuity of our consciousness based on recent scientific research on near-death experience in survivors of cardiac arrest.' Lecture for the IANDS Conference, 9 September at Virginia Beach, US.

van Lommel, P. (2010) *Consciousness Beyond Life: The Science of the Near-Death Experience.* New York, NY: Harper One.

Chapter 2

Corazza, O. and Schifano, F. (2010) 'Ketamine use: near-death states reported in a sample of 50 misusers.' *Substance Use and Misuse, 45,* 916–24.

Delgado-Rodriguez, M. and Llorca, J. (2004) 'Bias.' *Journal of Epidemiology and Community Health 58,* 635–641.

Fracasso, C., Aleyasin, S.E., Friedman, H. and Young, M.S. (2010) 'Near-Death Experiences among a Sample of Iranian Muslims.' *Journal of Near-Death Studies 29,* 265–272.

Gordis, L. (2008) *Epidemiology.* Fourth edition. Philadelphia, PA: Saunders.

Greyson, B. (1983) 'The Near-Death Experience Scale: construction, reliability, and validity.' *Journal of Nervous and Mental Disease 171,* 369–375.

Greyson, B. (1998) 'The incidence of near-death experiences.' *Medicine Psychiatry 1,* 92–99.

Greyson, B. (2003a) 'Incidence and correlates of near-death experiences in a cardiac care unit.' *General Hospital Psychiatry 25,* 269–276.

Greyson, B. (2003b) 'Near-death experiences in a Psychiatric Outpatient Clinic Population.' *Psychiatric Services 54,* 1649–1651.

Greyson, B., Holden, J.M. and Mounsey, J.P. (2006) 'Failure to elicit Near-Death Experiences in Induced Cardiac Arrest.' *Journal of Near-Death Studies 25,* 85–97.

Klemenc-Ketis, Z., Kersnik, J. and Grmec, S. (2010) 'The effect of carbon dioxide on near-death experiences in out-of-hospital cardiac arrest survivors: a prospective observational study.' *Critical Care 14* (R56).

Knoblauch, H., Schmied, I. and Schnettler, B. (2001) 'Different kinds of near-death experiences: a report on a survey in Germany.' *Journal of Near-Death Studies 20,* 15–29.

Kupuppuarchchi, K.A.L.A., Gambheera, H., Padmasekara, G. and Perera, M. (2008) 'Near-Death Experiences in suicide attempters in Sri Lanka.' *Journal of Near-Death Studies 26,* 295–301.

Lai, C.F., Kao, T.W., Wu, M.S., Chiang, S.S., *et al.* (2010) 'Impact of near-death experiences on dialysis patients: a multicentre collaborative study.' *American Journal of Kidney Diseases 50,* 124–132.

Moody, R.A. (1975) *Life After Life.* Atlanta, GA: Mockingbird Books.

Olson, M. and Dulaney, P. (1993) 'Life satisfaction, life review, and near-death experiences in the elderly.' *Journal of Holistic Nursing 11,* 368–382.

Parnia, S., Waller, D.G., Yeates, R. and Fenwick, P. (2001) 'A qualitative and quantitative study of the incidence, features and aetiology of near-death experiences in cardiac arrest survivors.' *Resuscitation 48,* 149–156.

Pasricha, S.K. (2008) 'Near-Death Experiences in India: prevalence and new features.' *Journal of Near-Death Studies 26,* 267–282.

Perera, M., Padmasekera, G. and Belanti, J. (2005) 'Prevalence of near-death experiences in Australia.' *Journal of Near-Death Studies 24,* 109–116.

Porta, M. and Last, J.M. (2008) *Dictionary of Epidemiology.* Fifth edition. Oxford: Oxford University Press.

Ring, K. (1980) *Life at Death. A Scientific Investigation of the Near-Death Experience.* New York, NY: Coward Mc-Cann & Geoghenan.

Schwaninger, J., Eisenberg, P.R., Schechtman, K.B. and Weiss, A.N. (2002) 'A prospective analysis of near-death experiences in cardiac arrest patients.' *Journal of Near-Death Studies 20,* 215–232.

van Lommel, P., van Wees, R., Meyers, V. and Elfferich, I. (2001) 'Near-Death experience in survivors of cardiac arrest: a prospective study in the Netherlands.' *The Lancet 358,* 2039–2045.

Chapter 3

American Psychiatric Association (2000) *Diagnostic and Statistical Manual of Mental Disorders*. Fourth edition. Text Revision. Washington, DC: American Psychiatric Association.

Atwater, P.M.H. (2007) *The Big Book of Near-Death Experiences: The Ultimate Guide To What Happens When We Die.* Charlottesville, VA: Hampton Roads Publishing Company, Inc.

Bates, B.C. and Stanley, A. (1985) 'The epidemiology and differential diagnosis of near-death experience.' *American Journal of Orthopsychiatry 55*, 542–549.

Blanke, O., Landis, T., Spinelli, L. and Seeck, M. (2004) 'Out-of-body experience and autoscopy of neurological origin.' *Brain 127*, 243–258.

Bush, N.E. (2009) 'Distressing Western Near-death Experiences: Finding a Way Through Abyss.' In J.M. Holden, B. Greyson and D. James (eds) *The Handbook of Near-Death Experiences: Thirty Years of Investigation.* Santa Barbara, California: Praeger Publishers.

Chesterman, L.P. and Boast, N. (1994) 'Multi-modal hallucinations.' *Psychopathology 27*, 273–280.

Devinsky, O. and Lai, G. (2008) 'Spirituality and religion in epilepsy.' *Epilepsy & Behavior 12*, 636–643.

Gabbard, G.O., Twemlow, S.W. and Jones, F.C. (1981) 'Do "near-death experiences" occur only near-death.' *Journal of Nervous and Mental Disease 169*, 374–377.

Greyson, B. (1983) 'The near-death experience scale: Construction, reliability, and validity.' *Journal of Nervous and Mental Disease 171*, 369–375.

Greyson, B. (1985) 'A typology of near-death experiences.' *American Journal of Psychiatry 142*, 967–969.

Greyson, B. (1990) 'Near-death encounters with and without near-death experiences: Comparative NDE scale profiles.' *Journal of Near-Death Studies 8*, 151–161.

Greyson, B. (2007) 'Consistency of near-death experience accounts over two decades: Are reports embellished over time?' *Resuscitation 73*, 407–411.

Greyson, B. and Bush, N.E. (1992) 'Distressing near-death experiences.' *Psychiatry 55*, 95–110.

Isaac, M. and Chand, P.K. (2006) 'Dissociative and conversion disorders: Defining boundaries.' *Current Opinion in Psychiatry 19*, 61–66.

Lange, R., Greyson, B. and Houran, J. (2004) 'A Rasch scaling validation of a "core" near-death experience.' *British Journal of Psychology 95*, 161–177.

Lishman, W. A. (1998) *Organic Psychiatry: The Psychological Consequences of Cerebral Disorder.* Third Edition. Carlton, Victoria: Blackwell Science.

Moody, R.A. (1975) *Life After Life.* Atlanta, GA: Mockingbird Books.

Noyes, R. and Kletti, R. (1976) 'Depersonalization in the face of life-threatening danger: An interpretation.' *Omega 7*, 103–114.

Perera, M., Padmasekara, G. and Belanti, J. (2005) 'Prevalence of near-death experiences in Australia.' *Journal of Near-Death Studies 24*, 109–116.

Reutens, S., Nielsen, O. and Sachdev, P. (2010) 'Depersonalisation disorder.' *Current Opinion in Psychiatry 23*, 278–283.

Ring, K. (1980) *Life at Death: A Scientific Investigation of the Near-Death Experience.* New York, NY: Coward, McCann & Geoghegan.

Rommer, B. (2000) *Blessing in Disguise: Another Side of The Near-Death Experience.* St Paul, MN: Llewellyn Publications.

Sabom, M.B. (1982) *Recollections of Death: A Medical Investigation.* New York, NY: Harper & Row.

van Lommel, P. (2010) *Consciousness Beyond Life: The Science of The Near-Death Experience.* New York, NY: Harper One.

van Lommel, P., van Wees, R., Meyers, V. and Elfferich, I. (2001) 'Near-death experience in survivors of cardiac arrest: a prospective study in the Netherlands.' *Lancet 358*, 2039–2045.

World Health Organization (1992) *The ICD-10 Classification of Mental and Behavioural Disorders: Clinical Descriptions and Diagnostic Guidelines.* Geneva: World Health Organization.

Chapter 4

Becker, C.B. (1981) 'The centrality of the near-death experience in Chinese pure land Buddhism.' *Anabiosis 1*, 154–171.

Belanti, J. Perera, M. and Jagadheesan, K. (2008) 'Phenomenology of near-death experiences: A cross cultural perspective.' *Transcultural Psychiatry 45*, 121–133.

Blackmore, S.J. (1982) *Beyond the Body: An Investigation of Out-of-the-Body Experiences.* London: Heinemann.

Blackmore, S.J. (1993) 'Near-death experiences in India: they have tunnels too.' *Journal of Near-Death Studies, 11*, 205–17.

Blackmore, S.J. and Troscianko, T. (1988) 'The physiology of the tunnel.' *Journal of Near-Death Studies 8*, 15–28.

Bullis D. (2005) *The Mahawamsa, The Great Chronicle of Sri Lanka* (originally written by Mahanama Thera in the fifth century AD). Colombo: Vijitha Yapa.

Carr, D. (1982) 'Pathophysiology of stress induced limbic lobe dysfunction: a hypothesis for NDEs.' *Journal of Near-Death Studies 2*, 75–89.

Corazza, O. (2008) *Near-Death Experiences: Exploring the Mind–Body Connection.* London/New York: Routledge.

Corazza, O. (2010) 'Exploring space-consciousness in near-death and other dissociative experiences.' *Journal of Consciousness Study.* Social Approaches to Consciousness II, Vol. 17, No 7–8.

Counts, D.A. (1983) 'Near-death and out-of-body experiences in a Melanesian society.' *Anabiosis 3*, 115–135.

Fenwick, P. and Fenwick, E. (1995) *The Truth in the Light: An Investigation of Over 300 Near-Death Experiences.* London: Headline.

Hadfield, P. (1991) 'Japanese find death a depressing experience.' *New Scientist 132*, 11.

Haraldsson, E. (2001) 'Some Recent Cases that I have Investigated in Sri Lanka.' In N. Senanayake (ed.) *Trends in Rebirth Research: Proceedings of an International Seminar.* Ratmalana: Sarvodaya Vishva Lekha.

Jayawardana, T. (2007) *Maranaya Abiyasa Asudutu Athdakeem.* Colombo: Sadeepa Publishing House.

Kellehear, A. (1993) 'Culture, biology and the near-death experience: a reappraisal.' *Journal of Nervous and Mental Disease 18*, 148–156.

Kellehear, A. (1996) *Experiencing Near-Death: Beyond Medicine and Religion.* Oxford: Oxford University Press.

Kellehear, A (2008) 'Census of non-western near-death experiences to 2005: Overview of the current data.' *Journal of Near-Death Studies 26*, 249–265.

Kuruppuarachchi, K.A.L.A., Gambheera, H., Padmasekara, G. and Perera, M. (2008) 'Near-death experiences in suicide attempters.' *Journal of Near-Death Studies 26*, 295–301.

Nishida, K. (1990) *An Inquiry into the Good.* (Translated from the original Japanese version by Masao Abe and Christopher Ives.) New Haven and London: Yale University Press.

Osis, K. and Haraldsson, E. (1977) *At the Hour of Death.* New York, NY: Avon.

Panditrao M.M., Singh, C. and Panditrao, M.M. (2010) 'An unanticipated cardiac arrest and unusual post-resuscitation psycho-behavioural phenomena/near-death experience in a patient with pregnancy induced hypertension and twin pregnancy undergoing elective lower segment caesarean section.' *Indian Journal of Anaesthesia 54*, 467–469.

Pasricha, S. and Stevenson, I. (1986) 'Near-death experiences in India: a preliminary report.' *Journal of Nervous and Mental Diseases 174*, 165–70.

Rahula, W. (2006) *What the Buddha Taught.* (First published in 1959.) Dehiwela: Buddhist Cultural Centre.

Rewathe-Thero (Rev), K. S. and Wijethilake, M.M. (2001) *Astral Body, Interim Existence and Mysterious Attraction.* (In Sinhalese, first published in 1998.) Colombo: Sadeepa Publishing House.

Rinpoche, S. (1992) *The Tibetan Book of the Living and the Dying.* London: Routledge.

Sotelo, J., Perez, R., Guevara, P. and Fernandez, A. (1985) 'Changes in brain, plasma and cerebrospinal fluid contents of B-endorphin in dogs at the moment of death.' *Neurological Research 17*, 223–225.

Story, F. (2000) *Rebirth as Doctrine and Experience: Essays and Case Studies.* Kandy: Buddhist Publication Society.

Sutherland, C. (1995) *Children of the Light.* Sydney: Bantam Books.

Tachibana, T. (1994) *Near-Death Experience.* Tokyo: Bungei Shunju. (Japanese only)

van Lommel, P., van Wees, R., Meyers, V. and Elfferich, I. (2001) 'Near-death experience in survivors of cardiac arrest: a prospective study in the Netherlands.' *Lancet 358,* 2039–2045.

Wickramasinghe, M. (2006a) *Aspects of Sinhala Culture.* Fifth Edition. Rajagiriya: Sarasa (Pvt) Ltd.

Wickramasinghe, M. (2006b) *Buddhism and Culture.* Third Edition. Rajagiriya: Sarasa (Pvt) Ltd.

Yamamura, H. (1998) '[Implications of Near-Death Experience for the Elderly in Terminal Care.]' *Nippon Ronen Igakkai Zasshi 35,* 103–115 (Abstract in English).

Zhi-ying, F. and Jian-Xun, L. (1992) 'The near-death experiences among survivors of the 1976 Tangshan Earthquake.' *Journal of Near-Death Studies 11,* 39–48.

Chapter 5

Atwater, P.M.H. (2003) *The New Children and Near-Death Experiences.* Rochester VT: Bear.

Bonenfant, R.J. (2001) 'A child's encounter with the devil: an unusual near-death experience with both blissful and frightening elements.' *Journal of Near-Death Studies 20,* 87–100.

Bonenfant, R. J. (2004) 'A comparative study of near-death experience and non-near-death experience outcomes in 56 survivors of clinical death.' *Journal of Near-Death Studies 22,* 155–178.

Bush, N.E. (1983) 'The near-death experience in children: shades of the prison house reopening.' *Anabiosis – The Journal for Near-Death Studies 3,* 177–193.

Bush, N.E. (2002) 'Afterward: making meaning after a frightening near-death experience.' *Journal of Near-Death Studies 21,* 99–133.

Colli, J.E., and Beck, T.E. (2003) 'Recovery from bulimia nervosa through near-death experience: a case study.' *Journal of Near-Death Studies 22,* 33–55.

Corcoran, D.K. (1988) 'Helping patients who've had near-death experiences.' *Nursing 18,* 34–39.

Enright, R. (2004) 'Silent journeys: the discovery of the near-death experience of a nonverbal adolescent.' *Journal of Near-Death Studies 22,* 195–208.

Fenwick, P. and Fenwick, E. (1995) *The Truth in the Light: An Investigation of Over 300 Near-Death Experiences.* London: Headline.

Flynn, C.P. (1986) *After the Beyond: Human Transformation and the Near-Death Experience.* Englewood Cliffs, NJ: Prentice-Hall.

Gabbard, G.O. and Twemlow, S.W. (1984) *With the Eyes of the Mind: An Empirical Analysis of Out-of-Body States.* New York, NY: Praeger.

Greyson, B. (1997) 'The near-death experience as a focus of clinical attention.' *Journal of Nervous and Mental Diseases 185,* 327–334.

Greyson, B. (2003) 'Incidence and correlates of near-death experiences on a cardiac care unit.' *General Hospital Psychiatry 25,* 269–276.

Herzog, D.B. and Herrin, J.T. (1985) 'Near-death experiences in the very young.' *Critical Care Medicine 13,* 1074–1075.

Hoffman, E. (1998) 'Peak experiences in childhood: An explanatory study.' *Journal of Humanistic Psychology 38,* 109–120.

Holden, J.M. and Joesten, L. (1990) 'Near-death veridicality research in the hospital setting: problems and promise.' *Journal of Near-Death Studies 9,* 45–54.

Horacek, B.J. (1997) 'Amazing grace: the healing effects of near-death experiences on those dying and grieving.' *Journal of Near-Death Studies 16,* 149–161.

Irwin, H. J. (1989) 'The near-death experience in childhood.' *Australian Parapsychological Review 14,* 7–11.

Kübler-Ross, E. (1983) *On Children and Death.* New York, NY: Macmillan.

Liester, M.B. (1998) 'Inner communications following the near-death experience.' *Journal of Near-Death Studies 16,* 233–248.

Manley, L.K. (1996) 'Enchanted journeys: near-death experiences and the emergency nurse.' *Journal of Emergency Nursing 22,* 311–316.

Moody, R.A. (1975) *Life After Life*. New York, NY: Bantam Books.

Morse, M.L. (1983) 'A near-death experience in a 7-year-old child.' *American Journal of Diseases of Children 137*, 959–961.

Morse, M., Conner, D. and Tyler, D. (1985) 'Near-death experiences in a pediatric population: A preliminary report.' *American Journal of Diseases of Children 139*, 595–600.

Morse, M., Castillo, P., Venecia, D., Milstein, J. and Tyler, D. C. (1986) 'Childhood near-death experiences.' *American Journal of Diseases of Children 140*, 1110–1114.

Morse, M.L. and Perry, P. (1990) *Closer to the Light: Learning from the Near-Death Experiences of Children*. New York, NY: Villard Books.

Morse, M.L. and Perry, P. (1992) *Transformed by the Light: The Powerful Effect of Near-Death Experiences on People's Lives*. New York, NY: Villard Books.

Morse, M.L. (1994a) 'Near-death experiences and death-related visions in children: Implications for the clinician.' *Current Problems in Pediatrics 24*, 55–83.

Morse, M.L. (1994b) 'Near-death experiences of children.' *Journal of Pediatric Oncology Nursing 11*, 139–144.

Parnia, S., Waller, D.G., Yeates, R. and Fenwick, P. (2001) 'A qualitative and quantitative study of the incidence, features and aetiology of near-death experiences in cardiac arrest survivors.' *Resuscitation 48*, 149–156.

Ring, K. (1982) *Life at Death: A Scientific Investigation of the Near-Death Experience*. New York, NY: Quill. (First published 1980.)

Ring, K. (1985) *Heading Toward Omega: In Search of the Meaning of the Near-Death Experience*. New York, NY: Quill. (First published 1984.)

Ring, K. (1992) *The Omega Project: Near-Death Experiences, UFO Encounters, and Mind at Large*. New York, NY: William Morrow and Company.

Ring, K. and Rosing, C. J. (1990) 'The Omega Project: An empirical study of the NDE-prone personality.' *Journal of Near-Death Studies 8*, 211–239.

Ring, K. and Valarino, E.E. (2000) *Lessons from the Light: What we can Learn from the Near-Death Experience*. Cambridge, MA: Moment Point Press.

Rosen, D.H. (1975) 'Suicide survivors: a follow-up study of persons who survived jumping from the Golden Gate and San Francisco-Oakland Bay Bridges.' *Western Journal of Medicine 122*, 289–294.

Sabom, M.B. (1982) *Recollections of Death: A Medical Investigation*. New York, NY: Harper and Row.

Schoenbeck, S.B. (1993) 'Exploring the mystery of near-death experiences.' *American Journal of Nursing 93*, 42–46.

Schwaninger, J., Eisenberg, P.R., Schechtman, K.B. and Weiss, A.N. (2002) 'A prospective analysis of near-death experiences in cardiac arrest patients.' *Journal of Near-Death Studies 20*, 215–232.

Serdahely, W.J. (1987–88) 'The near-death experience: Is the presence always the higher self?' *Omega 18*, 129–134.

Serdahely, W.J. (1989–90) 'A pediatric near-death experience: Tunnel variants.' *Omega 20*, 55–62.

Serdahely, W.J. (1990) 'Pediatric near-death experiences.' *Journal of Near-Death Studies 9*, 33–39.

Serdahely, W.J. (1991) 'A comparison of retrospective accounts of childhood near-death experiences with contemporary pediatric near-death experience accounts.' *Journal of Near-Death Studies 9*, 219–224.

Serdahely, W.J. (1992) 'Similarities between near-death experiences and multiple personality disorder.' *Journal of Near-Death Studies 11*, 19–38.

Serdahely, W.J. (1993) 'Near-death experiences and dissociation: Two cases.' *Journal of Near-Death Studies 12*, 85–94.

Serdahely, W. J. and Walker, B.A. (1990a) 'The near-death experience of a nonverbal person with congenital quadriplegia.' *Journal of Near-Death Studies 9*, 91–96.

Serdahely, W. J. and Walker, B.A. (1990b) 'A near-death experience at birth.' *Death Studies 14*, 177–183.

Shears, D., Elison, S., Garralda, M.E. and Nadel, S. (2002) 'Near-death experiences with meningococcal disease.' *Journal of the American Academy of Child and Adolescent Psychiatry 44*, 630–631.

Steiger, B. and Steiger, S.H. (1995) *Children of the Light: The Startling and Inspiring Truth about Children's Near-Death Experiences and how they Illumine the Beyond.* New York, NY: Signet.

Sutherland, C. (1991) 'The near-death experience: A nursing response.' *Pallicom 10,* 8–14.

Sutherland, C. (1992) *Transformed by the Light: Life After Near-Death Experiences.* Sydney, Australia: Bantam Books.

Sutherland, C. (1993) *Within the Light.* Sydney, Australia: Bantam Books.

Sutherland, C. (1995) *Children of the Light: The Near-Death Experiences of Children.* Sydney, Australia: Bantam Books.

Sutherland, C. (1997) *Beloved Visitors: Parents Tell of After-Death Visits from their Children.* Sydney, Australia: Bantam Books.

van Lommel, P., van Wees, R., Meyers, V. and Elfferich, I. (2001) 'Near-death experience in survivors of cardiac arrest: A prospective study in the Netherlands.' *Lancet 358,* 2039–2045.

Chapter 6

Blanke, O., Ortigue, S., Landis, T. and Seeck, M. (2002) 'Stimulating illusory own-body perceptions: The part of the brain that can induce out-of-body experiences has been located.' *Nature 419,* 269–270.

Blanke, O., Landis, T., Spinelli, L. and Seeck, M. (2004) 'Out-of-body experience and autoscopy of neurological origin.' *Brain 127,* 243–258.

Branston, N.M., Ladds, A., Symon, L. and Wang, A.D. (1984) 'Comparison of the effects of ischaemia on early components of the somatosensory evoked potential in brainstem, thalamus, end cerebral cortex.' *Journal of Cerebral Blood Flow and Metabolism 4,* 68–81.

Britton, W.B. and Bootzin, R.R. (2004) 'Near-death experiences and the temporal lobe.' *American Psychological Society 15,* 254–258.

Clute, H. and Levy, W.J. (1990) 'Electroencephalographic changes during brief cardiac arrest in humans.' *Anesthesiology 73,* 821–825.

de Vries, J.W., Bakker, P.F.A., Visser, G.H., Diephuis, J.C. and van Huffelen, A.C. (1998) 'Changes in cerebral oxygen uptake and cerebral electrical activity during defibrillation threshold testing.' *Anesthesia and Analgesia 87,* 16–20.

Gopalan, K.T., Lee, J., Ikeda, S. and Burch, C.M. (1999) 'Cerebral blood flow velocity during repeatedly induced ventricular fibrillation.' *Journal of Clinical Anesthesia 11,* 290–295.

Greyson, B. (2003) 'Incidence and correlates of near-death experiences in a cardiac care unit.' *General Hospital Psychiatry 25,* 269–276.

Grof, S. and Halifax, J. (1977) *The Human Encounter with Death.* New York, NY: Dutton.

Gua, J., White, J.A. and Batjer, H.H. (1995) 'Limited protective effects of etomidate during brainstem ischemia in dogs.' *Journal of Neurosurgery 82,* 278–284.

James, W. (1958) *The Varieties of Religious Experience: A Study in Human Nature.* New York: Mentor Books.

Jansen, K. (1996) 'Neuroscience, Ketamine and the Near-Death Experience: The Role of Glutamate and the NMDA-Receptor.' In L.W. Bailey and J. Yates (eds) *The Near-Death Experience: A Reader.* New York and London: Routledge.

Kelly, E.D. and Williams Kelly, E. (2007) *Irreducible Mind: Toward a Psychology for the 21st Century.* (Chapter 6: 'Unusual Experiences Near-Death and Related Phenomena.') Lanham: Rowman & Littlefield Publishers, Inc.

Klemenc-Ketis, Z., Kersnik, J. and Gremc, S. (2010) 'The effect of carbon dioxide on near-death experiences in out-of-hospital arrest survivors: a prospective observational study.' *Critical Care 14,* R56.

Kolar M., Krizmaric, M., Klemen, P. and Gremc, S. (2008) 'Partial pressure of end-tidal carbon dioxide successful predicts cardiopulmonary resuscitation in the field: A prospective observational study.' *Critical Care 12,* R115.

Lempert, T., Bauer, M. and Schmidt, D. (1994) 'Syncope and Near-Death Experience.' *Lancet 344,* 829–830.

Long, J. and Holden, J.M. (2007) 'Does the arousal system contribute to near-death and out-of-body experiences? A summary and response.' *Journal of Near-Death Studies 25,* 135–169.

Losasso, T.J., Muzzi, D.A., Meyer, F.B. and Sharbrough, F.W. (1992) 'Electroencephalographic monitoring of cerebral function during asystole and successful cardiopulmonary resuscitation.' *Anesthesia and Analgesia 75*, 12–19.

Mayer, J. and Marx, T. (1972) 'The Pathogenesis of EEG Changes during Crebral Anoxia.' In E. van der Drift (ed.) *Cardiac and Vascular Diseases/Handbook of Electroencephalography and Clinical Neurophysiology*, Vol. 14A, part A, pp. 5–11. Amsterdam: Elsevier.

Meduna, L.T. (1950) *Carbon Dioxide Therapy: A Neuropsychological Treatment of Nervous Disorders.* Springfield: Charles C. Thomas.

Nelson, K.R., Mattingly, M., Lee, S.A. and Schmitt, F.A. (2006) 'Does the arousal system contribute to near-death experience?' *Neurology 66*, 1003–1009.

Parnia, S. and Fenwick, P. (2002) 'Near-death experiences in cardiac arrest: visions of a dying brain or visions of a new science of consciousness.' *Resuscitation 52*, 5–11.

Parnia, S., Waller, D.G., Yeates, R. and Fenwick, P. (2001) 'A qualitative and quantitative study of the incidence, features and aetiology of near-death experience in cardiac arrest survivors.' *Resuscitation 48*, 149–156.

Penfield, W. (1958) *The Excitable Cortex in Conscious Man.* Liverpool: Liverpool University Press.

Penfield, W. (1975) *The Mystery of the Mind.* Princeton: Princeton University Press.

Penfield, W. (1955) 'The role of the temporal cortex in certain psychical phenomena.' *Journal of Mental Science* 101, 451–465.

Rodin, E. (1989) 'Comments on a neurobiological model for near-death experiences.' *Journal of Near-Death Studies 7*, 255–259.

Sanders, A.B., Kern, K.B., Otto, C.W., Milander, M.M. and Ewy, G.A. (1989) 'End-tidal carbon dioxide monitoring during cardiopulmonary resuscitation. a prognostic indicator for survival.' *Journal of the American Medical Association 262*, 1347–1351.

Sartori, P. (2006) 'The incidence and phenomenology of near-death experiences.' *Network Review (Scientific and Medical Network) 90*, 23–25.

Strassman, R. (2001) *DMT: The Spirit Molecule: A Doctors Revolutionary Research into the Biology of Near-Death and Mystical Experiences.* Vermont: Park Street Press.

Van Lommel, P. (2010) *Consciousness beyond Life. The Science of the Near-Death Experience.* New York: Harper Collins Publishers.

Van Lommel, P., Van Wees, R., Meyers, V., and Elfferich, I. (2001) 'Near-death experience in survivors of cardiac arrest: A prospective study in the Netherlands.' *The Lancet 358*, 2039–2045.

Whinnery, J.E. and Whinnery, A.M. (1990) 'Acceleration-induced loss of consciousness.' *Archives of Neurology 47*, 764–776.

Chapter 7

Bauer, M. (1985) 'Near-death experiences and attitude change.' *Anabiosis: Journal of Near-Death Studies, 5*, 39–47.

Bede (1975) *Ecclesiastical History of the English Nation.* London: Dent.

Blackmore, S. (1983) 'Birth and the OBE: an unhelpful analogy.' *Journal of American Society for Psychical Research 77*, 29–238.

Blackmore, S.J. (1993) 'Near-death experiences in India: they have tunnels, too.' *Journal of Near-Death Studies, 11*, 205–217.

Flynn, C.P. (1982) 'Meanings and implications of NDEr transformations: some preliminary findings and implications.' *Anabiosis: Journal of Near-Death Studies, 2*, 3–14.

Gabbard, G.O. and Twemlow, S.W. (1984) *With the Eyes of the Mind: An Empirical Analysis of Out-of-Body States.* New York, NY: Praeger.

Gabbard, G.O., Twemlow, S.W. and Jones, F. (1982) 'Differential diagnosis of altered mind-body perception.' *Psychiatry, 45*, 361–369.

Greyson, B. (1983) 'Near-death experiences and personal values.' *American Journal of Psychiatry, 140*, 618–620.

Greyson, B. (1992) 'Reduced death threat in near-death experiencers.' *Death Studies, 16*, 523–536.

Greyson, B. and Bush, N.E. (1992) 'Distressing near-death experiences.' *Psychiatry 55*, 1, 95–110.

Greyson, B. (1997) 'The near-death experience as a focus of clinical attention.' *Journal of Nervous and Mental Disease, 185*, 327–334.

Greyson, B. (2001) 'Posttraumatic stress symptoms following near-death experiences.' *American Journal of Orthopsychiatry*, 71, 368–373.

Greyson, B. and Stevenson, I (1980) 'The phenomenology of near-death experiences.' *American Journal of Psychiatry, 137*, 1193–1196.

Hazra, R.C. (1975) *Studies in the Puranic Records on Hindu Rites and Customs.* Delhi: Motilal Banarsidass. (Original work published 1940.)

Irwin, H.J. (1985) *Flight of Mind: A Psychological Study of the Out-of-Body Experience.* Metuchen, NJ: Scarecrow Press.

Kellehear, A. (2008) 'Census of non-Western NDEs to 2005: overview of the current data.' *Journal of Near-Death Studies, 26*, 249–265.

Kellehear, A., Stevenson, I., Pasricha, S. and Cook, E. (1994) 'The absence of tunnel sensation in near-death experiences from India.' *Journal of Near-Death Studies, 13*, 109–113.

Locke, T.P. and Schontz, F.C. (1983) 'Personality correlates of the near-death experience: a preliminary study.' *Journal of the American Society for Psychical Research, 77*, 311–318.

Moor, E. (1968) *The Hindu Pantheon.* Varanasi and Delhi: Indological Book House. (Original work published 1809.)

Murphy, T. (2001) 'Near-death experiences in Thailand.' *Journal of Near-Death Studies 19*, 161–178.

Noyes, R. (1980) 'Attitude change following near-death experiences.' *Psychiatry, 43*, 234–242.

Noyes, R. and Kletti, R. (1976) 'Depersonalization in the face of life-threatening danger: An interpretation.' *Omega 7*, 103–114.

Osis, K. and Haraldsson, E. (1977) *At the Hour of Death.* New York, NY: Avon Books.

Pasricha, S. (1993) 'A systematic survey of NDEs in South India.' *Journal of Scientific Exploration, 7*, 161–171.

Pasricha, S.K. (1995) 'Near-death experiences in South India: A systematic survey.' *Journal of Scientific Exploration, 9*, 79–88.

Pasricha, S.K. (2008) 'Near-death experiences in India: Prevalence and new features.' *Journal of Near-Death Studies, 26*, 267–282.

Pasricha, S. and Stevenson, I. (1986) 'Near-death experiences in India: A preliminary report.' *Journal of Nervous and Mental Disease, 174*, 165–170.

Ring, K. (1980) *Life at Death: A Scientific Investigation of the Near-Death Experience.* New York, NY: Coward, McCann.

Sabom, M.B. (1982) *Recollections of Death: A Medical Investigation.* New York, NY: Harper & Row.

Sagan, C. (1979) *Broca's Brain: Reflections on the Romance of Science.* New York, NY: Random House.

Walker, B. (1983) *Hindu World: An Encyclopedia Survey of Hinduism.* (2 vols.) New Delhi: Munshiram Manoharlal Publishers. (First published in 1968.)

Wilkins, W.J. (1978) *Hindu Mythology: Vedic and Puranic.* Delhi: Rupa and Co. (First published in 1882.)

Chapter 8

Atwater, P.M.H. (2009) *Beyond The Light.* Kill Devil Hills, NC: Transpersonal Publishing.

Bose, S.N. (1924) 'Plancks Gesetz und Lichtquantenhypothese.' *Zeitschrift für Physik 26*, 178.

Chalmers, D.J. (1995) 'Facing up to the problem of consciousness.' *Journal of Consciousness Studies 2*, 200–219.

Chen, L.-H. (2007) 'What is the soul, but a humble pineal gland.' *New Scientist* Dec 15–21.

Coles, M.G.H. and Rugg, M.D. (1996) 'Event related brain potentials: an introduction.' *Electrophysiology of Mind.* Oxford Scholarship Online Monographs. pp.1–27.

Department of Youth Services. Available at www.dys.ohio.gov/dnn/Home/tabid/36/Default.aspx. Accessed 11 February 2011.

Fenwick, P. and Fenwick, E. (1995) *The Truth in the Light.* London: Headline.

Hecht, S. and Verrijp, C.D. (1933) 'Intermittent stimulation by light. II. The relation between intensity and critical fusion frequency for different retinal locations.' *Journal of General Physiology 17*, 251–265.

Hirano, I. and Hirai, N. (1986) 'Holography in the single photon region.' *Applied Optics 25*, 1741–1742.

Kvaerne, P. (2001) *The Bon Religion of Tibet: The Iconography of a Living Tradition.* Boston: Shambhala.

Laszlo, E. (2007) *Science and the Akashic Field.* Vermont: Inner Traditions.

Liberles, S.D. (2009) 'Trace amine-associated receptors are olfactory receptors in vertebrates.' *Annals of the New York Academy of Sciences 1170*, 168–72.

Mavromatis, A. (2010) *Hypnagogia: The Unique State of Consciousness Between Wakefulness and Sleep.* Third Edition. London: Thyrsos Press.

Meissl, H. and Yanez, J. (1994) 'Pineal photosensitivity: A comparison with retinal photoreception.' *Acta Neurobiologiae Experimentalis 54*, 19–21.

Moller, M. and Baeres, F.M.M. (2002) 'The anatomy and innervation of mammalian pineal gland.' *Cell Tissue Research 309*, 139–150.

Moody, R.A. (1975) *Life After Life.* Covington, GA: Mockingbird Books.

Moody, R.A. (1988) *The Light Beyond.* New York, NY: Bantam Books.

Pandi-Perumal, S.R., Srinivasan, V., Maestroni, G.J., Cardinali, D.P., Poeggeler, B. and Hardeland, R. (2006) 'Melatonin: nature's most versatile biological signal?' *Federation of European Biological Societies Journal 273*, 2813–2838.

Regan, D. (1989) *Human Brain Electrophysiology: Evoked Potentials and Evoked Magnetic Fields in Science and Medicine.* New York, NY: Elsevier.

Ring, K. and Elsaesser-Valarino, E. (2000) *Lessons From The Light.* Needham, MA: Moment Point Press.

Stahl, S.M. (2000) *Essential Psychopharmacology: Neuroscientific Basis and Practical Applications.* Second Edition. Port Melbourne, Victoria: Cambridge University Press.

Steele, B. (2009) 'Frozen helium-4 may be an unusual "superglass".' Available at www.physorg.com/news160408487.html. Accessed on 14 February 2011.

Stehle, J.H., Sassde, A., Rawashdeh, O., Ackermann, K., Jilg, A., Sebesteny, T. and Maronde, E. (2011) 'A survey of molecular details in the human pineal gland in the light of phylogeny, structure, function and chronobiological diseases.' *Journal of Pineal Research 50*, 4, 1–27

Strassman, R. (2001) *DMT: The Spirit Molecule: A Doctor's Revolutionary Research into the Biology of Near-Death and Mystical Experiences.* Victoria: Brumby Books and Music.

Vivien-Roels, B. and Humbert, W. (1977) 'The lipopigments of the pineal gland of Testudo hemanni (Reptile, Chelonian): microprobe analysis and physiological significance.' *Journal of Ultrastructure Research 61*, 134–139.

Winkler, E. *The Elias Project.* Available at http://users.telenet.be/limen/ndeurope/articles/artelias.html. Accessed on 14 February 2011.

Winkler, E (2007) *Erleuchtung Im Augenblick Des Todes.* Norderstedt, Germany: BOD.

Chapter 9

Armstrong, K. (1991) *Muhammad.* London: Gollancz.

Armstrong, K. (1993) *A History of God.* London: Heinemann, 1993 (see p.163 for citation from Jalal al-Din Suyiti, al-itqan fi'ulum al-aq'ran).

Ayer, A.J. (1988) 'What I saw when I was dead.' *Sunday Telegraph,* 28 August. (Re-presented in Edwards, P. (1992) *Immortality.* New York, Macmillan.)

Badham, P. (1976) *Christian Beliefs about Life After Death.* London: MacMillan..

Bukyo Dendo Kyokai (1980) *The Teaching of Buddha.* Tokyo: Buddhist Promoting Foundation.

Cohn-Sherbok, D. (1987) 'Death and Immortality in the Jewish Tradition.' In P. Badham and L. Badham (eds) *Death and Immortality in the Religions of the World.* New York, NY: Paragon.

Evans-Wentz, W.Y. (1957) *The Tibetan Book of the Dead or the After-Death Experiences on the Bardo Plane, according to Lama Kazi Dawa-Sumdup's English Rendering.* New York, NY: Oxford University Press. (First published in 1927.)

Hick, J. (1976) *Death and Eternal Life.* London: Macmillan.

Hick, J. (1983) *The Second Christianity.* London: SCM.

Neuner, J. and Dupuis, J. (1983) *The Christian Faith in the Doctrinal Documents of the Catholic Church.* London: Collins.

Plato (1955 edition) *The Republic.* Translated by H.D.P. Lee. Harmondsworth: Penguin.

Rimpoche, S. (1992) *The Tibetan Book of Living and Dying.* London: Routledge.

Shushan, G. (2009) *Conceptions of the Afterlife in Early Civilizations.* London and New York: Continuum International Publishing.

St John of the Cross (1957) *The Dark Night of the Soul.* Bk.2 Ch.24. Translated by K. Reinhardt. London: Constable.

St. John of the Cross (1960) *Poems.* Translated by R.Campbell. Baltimore: Penguin.

St Paul (1989) 'Second Letter to the Corinthians.' *The Revised English Bible.* Oxford and Cambridge University Presses.

Cox-Chapman, M. (1996) *Glimpses of Heaven: The Near-Death Experience.* London: Hale.

Chapter 10

Fenwick, P. and Fenwick, E. (2008) *The Art of Dying.* London: Continuum.

Fenwick, P. and Fenwick, E. (1995) *The Truth in the Light.* London: Headline.

Fenwick, P., Lovelace, H. and Brayne, S. (2009) 'Comfort for the dying: five year retrospective and one year prospective studies of end of life experiences.' *Archives of Gerontology and Geriatrics, 51*, 2, 173–179.

Greyson, B. (1983) 'Near-death experience scale: construction, reliability and validity.' *Journal of Nervous and Mental Disease 171*, 6, 369–75.

Greyson, B. (1992–93) 'Near-death experiences and anti-suicidal attitudes.' *Omega 26*, 81–89.

Greyson, B. and Bush, N.E. (1992) 'Distressing near-death experiences.' *Psychiatry 55*, 95–110.

Greyson, B. and Ring, K. (2004) 'The Life change inventory – revised.' *Journal of Near-Death Studies 23*, 41–54.

Noyes, R., Fenwick, P., Holden, J. and Christian, S. (2009) 'After-effects of Pleasurable Western Adult Near-Death Experiences.' In J. Holden, B. Greyson and D. James (eds) *The Handbook of Near-death Experiences: Thirty years of Investigation.* Oxford: Praeger.

Sutherland, C. (1989) 'Psychic phenomena following near-death experiences: an Australian study.' *Journal of Near-Death Studies 8*, 93–102

Sutherland, C. (1992) *Transformed by the Light: Life After Death Experiences.* New York, NY: Bantam Books.

Twemlow, S. and Gabbard, G. (1984–5) 'The influence of demographic/psychological factors and pre-existing conditions on the near-death experience.' *Omega 15*, 223–35.

van Lommel, P., van Wees, R., Meyers, V. and Elferich, I. (2001) 'Near death experiences in survivors of cardiac arrest: a prospective study in the Netherlands.' *Lancet 358*, 2039–2045.

Chapter 11

Brocki, J.M. and Wearden, A.J. (2006) 'A critical evaluation of the use of interpretative phenomenological analysis (IPA) in health psychology.' *Psychology & Health, 21*, 1, 87–108.

Braithwaite, J.J. (2008) 'Towards a cognitive neuroscience of the dying brain.' *The [UK] Skeptic 21*, 2, 8–16.

Braud, W. (1993) 'Honoring our natural experiences.' *Journal of the American Society for Psychical Research 88*, 3, 293–308.

Fenwick, P. and Fenwick, E. (1995) *The Truth in the Light.* London: Headline.

Greyson, B. (1983) 'The Near-Death Experience Scale.' *Journal of Nervous and Mental Disease, 171*, 6, 369–375.

Greyson, B. (2000) 'Near-Death Experiences.' In E. Cardeña, S.J. Lynn and S.C. Krippner (eds) *Varieties of Anomalous Experience: Examining the Scientific Evidence.* Washington, DC: American Psychological Association.

Hufford, D. (1982) *The Terror That Comes in the Night: An Experience-Centered Study of Supernatural Assault Traditions.* Philadelphia, PA: University of Pennsylvania Press.

Lundahl, C.R. (1993) 'The near-death experience: A theoretical summarization.' *Journal of Near-Death Studies, 12,* 105–118.

McClenon, J. (1991) 'Social scientific paradigms for investigating anomalous experience.' *Journal of Scientific Exploration, 5,* 2, 191–203.

McClenon, J. (2010) 'Near-Death Experiences, Out-of-Body Experiences and Social Scientific Paradigms.' In C.D. Murray (ed.) *Psychological Scientific Perspectives on Out-of-Body and Near-Death Experiences.* New York, NY: Nova Science Publishers, Inc.

Moody, R.A. (1975) *Life After Life.* Covington, GA: Mockingbird Books.

Moody, R.A. (1977) *Reflections on Life After Life.* St. Simon's Island, GA: Mockingbird Books.

Morris, L.L. and Knafl, K. (2003) 'The nature and meaning of the near-death experience for patients and critical care nurses.' *Journal of Near-Death Studies, 21,* 139–167.

Murray, C.D. (2010) *Psychological Scientific Perspectives on Out-of-Body and Near-Death Experiences.* New York, NY: Nova Science Publishers, Inc.

Noyes, R. (1972) 'The experience of dying.' *Psychiatry, 35,* 174–184.

Palmer, J. (2010) 'Out-of-Body and Near-Death Experiences as Evidence for Externalization or Survival.' In C.D. Murray (ed.) (2010) *Psychological Scientific Perspectives on Out-of-Body and Near-Death Experiences.* New York, NY: Nova Science Publishers, Inc.

Parnia, S., Waller, D.G., Yeates, R. and Fenwick, P. (2001) 'A qualitative and quantitative study of the incidence, features and aetiology of near-death experiences in cardiac arrest survivors.' *Resusitation 48,* 149–156.

Perera, M., Padmasekara, G. and Belanti, J. (2005) 'Prevalence of near-death experiences in Australia.' *Journal of Near-Death Studies 24,* 109–116.

Roe, C.A. (2001) 'Near-Death Experiences.' In R. Roberts and D. Groome (eds) *Parapsychology: The Science of Unusual Experience.* London: Arnold.

Sartori, P. (2008) *The Near-Death Experiences of Hospitalized Intensive Care Patients: A Five Year Clinical Study.* Lampeter, Ceredigion: The Edwin Mellen Press.

Schwartz, E.K. (1949) 'The Study of Spontaneous Psi Experiences.' *Journal of the American Society for Psychical Research, 43,* 125–136.

van Lommel, P., van Wees, R., and Meyers, V. (2001) 'Near-death experiences in survivors of cardiac arrest: A prospective study in the Netherlands.' *The Lancet 358,* 2039–2045.

White, R.A. (1997) 'Dissociation, Narrative, and Exceptional Human Experience.' In S. Krippner and S. Powers (eds) *Broken Images, Broken Selves: Dissociative Narratives in Clinical Practice.* Washington, DC: Brunner-Mazel.

Wilde, D. and Murray, C.D. (2010) 'Interpreting the anomalous: Finding meaning in out-of-body and near-death experiences'. *Qualitative Research in Psychology 7,* 1, 57–72.

Suggested reading

Greyson, B. (1997) 'The near-death experience as a focus of clinical attention.' *Journal of Nervous and Mental Disease 185,* 5, 327–334.

Greyson, B. (2000) 'Near-Death Experiences.' In E. Cardeña, S. J. Lynn and S. C. Krippner (eds) *Varieties of Anomalous Experience: Examining the Scientific Evidence.* Washington, DC: American Psychological Association.

Morris, L.L. and Knafl, K. (2003) 'The nature and meaning of the near-death experience for patients and critical care nurses.' *Journal of Near-Death Studies 21,* 3, 139–167.

Murray, C.D. (2010) *Psychological Scientific Perspectives on Out-of-Body and Near-Death Experiences.* New York: Nova Science Publishers, Inc.

Smith, J.A., Flowers, P. and Larkin, M. (2009) *Interpretative Phenomenological Analysis: Theory, Method and Research.* London: Sage.

Wilde, D. and Murray, C.D. (2009) 'The evolving self: finding meaning in near-death experiences using interpretative phenomenological analysis.' *Mental Health, Religion & Culture 12,* 3, 223–239.

Wilde, D. and Murray, C.D. (2010) 'Interpreting the anomalous: finding meaning in out-of-body and near-death experiences.' *Qualitative Research in Psychology 7,* 1, 57–72.

Subject Index

Italic page numbers indicate tables.

aetiology 28
affect 69
after-effects 21–2, 41–2, 72–3, 100, 122–4, 125–6
Akashic Record 113
amines 114–15
amnesia 33–4
angelic presence 70
antecedent events 20–1
applied research 128–9
assessment 25–8, 121
Association for the Scientific Study of Near-Death Phenomena 18
Astral body 60
At the Hour of Death 55
atheism 120
Atman 60
Austria 104–7
autoscopy 99–100
Axelrod, Julius 114–15

Bardo 108
Being of Light 120–1
belief systems, effect of 62
bereavement 74
Beyond the Light 103
biological bases 15
birth memory 98–9
Bön 107–8, 111
Bose-Einstein Condensation 112–13
Bose, Satyendra Nath 112
brain
    chemical reactions 84–5
    and consciousness 90–1, 111
    electrical activity 86–7
    function during cardiac arrest 91–2
brain damage 126
Buddhism 57, 60, 107, 119

carbon-dioxide overload 83–4
cardiac arrest, brain function 91–2
cardiac arrest study 89–90
Catholicism 121

Chamberlain, D.B. 67–8
Chang Tsai 112
chemical reactions in brain 84–5
ch'i 112, 113
children
    antecedent events 21
    compensation and integration 22
    content of NDEs 69–73
    experiences 14
    helping 74–7
    overview 63–4
    summary and conclusions 77
    telling others 75–6
China 52
Chinese original quiet sitting 110–11
Christianity 118–19
circumstances, of NDEs 19, 68–9, *81*
classical model 19–20
Clear Light of Death 107–8
Clear Light of Sleep 108
clinical tests, need for 22
clinicians, advice to 101–2
close to death experiences 123–4
Closer to the Light 64
cognitive abilities 21
cognitive structures, common to cultures 61–2
coherent light 113
cohort studies 25, 28–9, 32
coming back 71
compensation and integration 22
conceptualization, of NDEs 25
Condition After Death 121
consciousness 19, 90–1, 111
control studies 28
cortical stimulation 86–7
cosmic consciousness 46–7
counselling 76, 101
cross-cultural aspects 51–2, 61–2
cross-sectional studies 25, 28, 31–2
cultural source theory 132
culture, effect of 60, 61, 62, 98–9
cumulative incidence 26

darkness to light 69–70
death anxiety, decline in 72
death, attitudes to 42, 74
death-bed coincidence 127
death-bed visions 58
delok 60, 119
depersonalization 43–4, 99
descriptive studies 28
Diagnostic and Statistical Manual of Mental Disorders, Fourth Edition, Text Revision (DSMIV- TR) 43, 44
diagnostic clarification 43–7
difference, feeling of 73
differential diagnosis 43–7
dimethyltryptamine (DMT) 45, 114–16
dissociation 44
distressing NDEs 39–40
drawing 76
Dream of Gerontius 121
Dream Yoga 107–9
drug-induced states 45
Dutugemunu 58
dying 74

early Israelite religion 117
ecstasy 118
eidetic essences 61–2
electrical activity in brain 86–7
electrical sensitivity 21
electroencephalogram (EEG) studies 88, 130–1
elements, of NDEs 19–20, 36, 81
Elias project 104–7
empathy 62
encounters, during NDEs 70
end-of-life experiences 15, 127
endorphin 84–5
enlightenment 107–8, 110–11
epidemiological data, lack of 129–30
epidemiological studies
    analytical studies 28–9
    criteria and questions for critical appraisal *30*
    critical appraisal 29–31
    descriptive studies 28
    design issues 31–4

errors 31
exclusion 32–3
future research 35
included in review 27
information bias 33–4
other design issues 34
overview 24–5
screening for candidates 35
selection bias 29, 30, 31–2
summary and conclusions 35
epidemiological techniques, use of 25
epilepsy 46, 86
evaluation, instruments for 47–9, 123
Event-Related Potential (ERP) 106
experimental studies 28
explanatory model 115–16
external validity 29

fear death experiences 123
fighter pilots 82
Flicker Fusion Threshold (FFT) 106
follow-up, loss to 32
future research 15
    after-effects 132
    applied research 128–9
    electroencephalogram (EEG) studies 130–1
    epidemiological studies 129–30
    lived experience 132–3
    need for consensus definition 129
    prospective studies 131
    qualitative 132–3
    when? of NDEs 130

Gallup Poll Survey 20
generalizability 29
Greyson, Bruce 12
grieving 74
group NDEs 14, 23

hallucinations 44–5
Haraldsson, Erlendur 108
healing 74
health care givers, attitude to reports of NDEs 13
health care professionals 75
Heisenberg Uncertainty Principle 112
hellish symbolism 40
Hinduism 119–20
holograms 113
hyperventilation 82
hypnagogia 108
hypnapompia 108

I Died Three Times in 1977 18
idiosyncracy 132
illusion 87
incidence 11, 26, 31
incidence studies 26–8
India 54–5
Indian cases 95–8
information bias 33–4
information, providing 76
integration 22
integration, of experience 22
intellect, enhancement 19
inter-rater bias 33
inter-rater reliability 33
Interim Existence 60
internal validity 29
International Association for Near-Death Studies (IANDS) 18, 135
Islam 119

Japan 52–4
Judaism 117–18
judgement 40

Kübler-Ross, Elisabeth 12

Lama Kazi Dawa-Samdup 120
lasers 113
leaving the body 69
Lessons from the Light 67, 103
Life After Life 17, 132
Life at Death 18
life review 40, 70
light
    coherent 113
    Dream Yoga 107–9
    Elias project 104–7
    moving towards 69–70
    overview 103–4
    Taiwan experiment 110–11
listening 62, 75–6
Lucia 107, 108–9, 115–16
Lucid Light Device 107, 108–9, 115–16
luminous presence 70
Lyh-Horng Chen 110–11

materialism 93
measure of disease frequency 25–6
measurement, difficulties of 35
medical model 15
medical schools 22
meditation 46–7, 110–11
Melanesia 58–60
melatonin 110
memory 67–8, 111–14
men, antecedent events 21
metabolic changes 21
mission, sense of 70

Moody, Raymond Jr 12, 17–18
moving from darkness to light 69–70
Muhammad 119

nature of experience 11–12
NDE Questionnaire 49
Near- Death Experience 53
Near-Death Experience Scale (NDES) 25, 33, 35, 48–9, 123
near-death experiences (NDEs)
    definition 19
    interest in 18
    major categories of 39–40
    summary and conclusions 135–7
negative NDEs 124
nested case control study 29
neuro-chemical bases 15
neurotransmitters 114–15
Night Journey 119
non-locality 92
non-response bias 32–3
non-Western studies 51–2, 60–2

observational studies 28–9
odd phenomena 72
operationalization, of NDEs 25
organic factors 124
originality 62
out-of-body experiences (OBE) 45–6, 69, 83, 87
oxygen deficiency 82–3

paradoxical sensation 40
parapsychological phenomena 72, 124–5
pathophysiology
    looking beyond 92–3
    overview 79–80
    summary and conclusions 93
    summary of theories 90–2
    theories 80–90
Perera, Mahendra 12–13
perinatal memory 67–8
period prevalence 26, 28
personal experience
    adults and children 64–5
    Barbara 66
    Carol Jean Morres 71
    Daniel 78
    David 76–7
    Dorothea 70
    Emily 73
    future research 132–3
    George Ritchie 17–18
    Hal 71
    Hannah 64–5, 66
    A.J. Ayer 120
    Japan 53–4

personal experience *cont.*
  John Belanti 37–9
  Katie 63–4
  Marcella 67
  Marja, 74
  Mark Botts 68
  Melanesia 58–60
  Mr A 42–3
  Mr M 97
  Mrs V. 96–7
  Mrs VN 97–8
  Natalie 70
  Sri Lanka 56–7
  Tommy 69
  unnamed infant 70
  Vasudev Pandey 54
  very young children 67–8
personal flashforward 70
personality changes 42
personality factors 125
phenomenology 36, 37–9,
  42–3, 49
physical experiences 11–12
physiological effects 21
physiological theories 82–4
pineal gland 109–11, 113, 115
place 61
pleasurable NDEs 39
point prevalence 26
populations of interest 29
post-traumatic stress disorder
  (PTSD) 100, 132
precognition 72
prevalence *see* incidence
Price, H.H. 119
Proeckl, Carola 106, 108
Proeckl, Dirk 106, 108–9, 115
progression 41
prospective cohort design 29
prospective studies 131
prototypical features 40
psychedelics 85
psychological aspects 15, 94–5,
  101–2
psychological changes 21
psychological effects 100
psychological interpretations
  98–100
psychopathological states 43–4
psychotherapy 101
publications, range of 13
Pure-land scriptures 120–1
Purusa 60

rapid eye movement (REM) 88
Rasch model 48
rates 26
ratios 26
reality 113
realness 61
reassurance 76

recall bias 29, 35, 65–6
reliability, of retrospective
  accounts 65–6
religion
  attitudes to 42
  Buddhism 57, 60, 107, 119
  Catholicism 121
  Christianity 118
  early Israelite 117
  Hinduism 119
  Islam 119
  Judaism 117–18
  Zoroastrianism 118
religious practices 15
religious significance 117–21
religious visions 55
REM intrusion 88
repeat episodes 34
repression, of experience 22
Republic 118
research, future of 15, 128–34
residual marks 95–6
responses, variations between
  children and adults 22
retrospective accounts, reliability
  65–6
retrospective studies 28–9
Ring, Kenneth 12

safe environment 62
scenario patterns 20
selection bias 29, 30, 31–2, 35
selective memory 33
sensations, heightened 21
sensitivity 72
shared NDEs 14, 22–3
signature features 49
similarities, cross-cultural 15
sleep disorders 88
spirituality 72
Sri Lanka 56–8
St Paul 118–19, 121
staging 41
suicide survivors 105
synaesthesia 21, 72

Taiwan experiment 110–11
talking 74
Tao 60
teenagers, content of NDEs
  69–73
telling others 71, 75
temporal lobe epilepsy (TLE) 46
The ICD-10 Classification of
  Mental and Behavioural
  Disorders Tenth Revision
  (ICD-10) 44
The Life Change Questionnaire
  123
The Light Beyond 103

The Near-Death Experience:
  Problems, Prospects,
  Perspectives 18
The Occidental Book of Death and
  Dying 106
The Tibetan Book of the Dead 118,
  119–20
The Truth in the Light 103
theories
  carbon-dioxide overload
  83–4
  of cause and content 80–90
  cortical stimulation 86–7
  EEG and sleep disorders 88
  endorphin 84–5
  ketamine 84
  oxygen deficiency 82–3
  psychedelics 85
  summary 90–2
therapists 62
time 61
touch 74–5
Trace Amine-Associated
  Receptors (TAARs) 115
transcendence 61
transcendent mystical
  experiences 123
transcendental meditation 46–7
transformation 62
treatment 126
2 Corinthians 118
typology 40–1

universality 62

Valsalva manoeuvre 82
value changes 42
value of experience 62
Visual Evoked Potential (VEP)
  106
volunteer bias 32

Weighted Core Experience Index
  (WCEI) Scale 25, 47–8
when? of NDEs 130
Winkler, Engelbert J. 104–7,
  108–9, 115
With the Eyes of the Mind 64
women, antecedent events 20–1

Zero Point Energy 111–13
Zero Point Field 112–13
Zohar 117–18
Zoroastrianism 118

Author Index

American Psychiatric Association 43–4
Armstrong, K. 119
Atwater, P.M.H. 14, 18, 21, 23, 40–1, 49, 71, 72, 103
Ayer, A.J. 120

Badham, P. 15, 117
Baeres, F.M.M. 110
Bates, B.C. 45, 46
Bauer, M. 82, 100
Beck, T.E. 68
Becker, C. 52
Bede 96
Belanti, J. 14, 32, 49, 61, 129
Blackmore, S. 54–5, 60, 96, 99
Blanke, O. 46, 87
Boast, N. 45
Bonenfant, R. 66, 72, 76
Bootzin, R.R. 88
Bose, S.N. 112
Braithwaite, J.J. 130
Branston, N.M. 91
Braud, W. 132
Brayne, S. 124, 127
Britton, W.B. 88
Brocki, J.M. 133
Bukyo Dendo Kyokai, 120–1
Bullis, D. 58
Bush, N.E. 39, 40, 64, 66, 67, 76, 124

Carr, D. 60
Castillo, P. 64
Chalmers, D. 111
Chand, P.K. 44
Chesterman, P.P. 45
Clute, H. 91
Cohn-Sherbok, D. 117
Coles, M.G.H. 106
Colli, J.E. 68
Conner, D. 64
Corazza, O. 14, 31, 53–4, 61
Corcoran, D.J. 75, 76
Counts, D.A. 58–60
Cox-Chapman, M. 118

De Vries, J.W. 91

Devinsky, O. 46
Dulaney, P. 25
Dupuis, J. 121

Elsaesser Valarino, E. 67–8, 103
Enright, R. 76–7
Evans-Wentz, W.Y. 118, 120

Fenwick, E. 53, 68, 72, 103, 123, 127, 130
Fenwick, P. 15, 53, 68, 72, 91, 103, 123, 127, 130
Flynn, C. 18, 73, 94, 100
Fracasso, C. 34

Gabbard, G. 45, 64, 66, 71, 94, 99, 125
Gallup, G. 20
Gopalan, K.T. 91
Gordis, L. 26, 29
Gremc, S. 32, 83–4
Greyson, B. 18, 25, 31, 32, 33, 34, 39, 40, 48, 49, 68, 73, 76, 90, 94, 100, 101, 123, 124, 126, 129
Grof, S. 85

Halifax, J. 85
Haraldsson, E. 55, 58, 95
Hata, Y. 53
Hecht, S. 106
Herrin, J.T. 64, 70
Herzog, D.B. 64, 70
Hick, J. 119
Hirai, A. 113
Hirano, I. 113
Hoffman, E. 68, 77–8
Holden, J. 68, 88
Horacek, B. 74
Houran, J. 48
Hufford, D. 132
Humbert, W. 110

International Association for Near-Death Studies (IANDS) 19
Irwin, H.J. 99
Isaac, M. 44

Jagadheesan, K. 14, 61
James, W. 79
Jansen, K. 84
Jayasuriya, R. 14
Jayawardana, T. 56, 58
Jian-Xun, L. 52
Joesten, L. 68
Jones, F. 45, 99

Kellehear, A. 51–2, 61, 96, 99
Kelly, E.D. 18, 92
Kersnik, J. 32, 83–4
Klemenc-Ketis, Z. 32, 33, 83–4
Kletti, R. 43, 99
Knafl, K. 133
Knoblauch, H. 31–2
Kolar, M. 84
Kübler-Ross, E. 17, 69
Kuruppuarachchi, K.A.L.A. 14, 56
Kvaerne, P. 107

Lai, C.F. 35
Lai, G. 46
Lange, R. 48
Last, J.M. 29
Laszlo, E. 112
Lempert, T. 82
Levy, W.J. 91
Liberles, S.D. 115
Lishman, W.A. 45, 46
Locke, T.P. 99
Long, J. 88
Losasso, T.J. 91
Lovelace, H. 127
Lundahl, C.R. 129

McClenon, J. 132
Manley, L.K. 74–5, 76
Marx, T. 91
Mavromatis, A. 108
Mayer, J. 91
Meduna, L.T. 83
Meissl, H. 109
Milstein, J. 64
Moller, M. 110

Moody, R.A. 17, 19, 20, 25, 31, 36, 39, 41, 49, 63, 72, 103, 129, 132
Morgan, D.H. 21
Morris, L.L. 133
Morse, M. 63–4, 66, 68, 72, 75, 76
Murphy, T. 99
Murray, C. 15, 130, 132

Nelson, K.R. 88
Neuner, J. 121
Nielsen, O. 44
Nishida, K. 60
Noyes, R. 43, 94, 99, 100, 123, 129

Olson, M. 25
Osis, K. 55, 95

Padmasekera, G. 32, 49, 129
Palmer, J. 130
Pandi-Perumal, S.R. 110
Panditrao, M.M. 55
Parnia, S. 33, 68, 90, 91, 131
Pasricha, S. 15, 32, 34, 35, 54, 60, 94, 95, 96, 99, 100
Peake, A. 15
Penfield, W. 87
Perera, M. 14, 32, 35, 49, 61, 129
Perry, P. 63–4, 68, 72
Plato 118
Porta, M. 29
Proctor, W. 20

Regan, D. 106
Reutens, S. 44
Rewathe-Thero, K.S. 60
Ring, K. 18, 25, 31, 41–2, 47, 67–9, 70, 72, 94, 100, 103, 123
Rinpoche, S. 60, 119
Ritchie, G. 17–18
Rodin, E. 86
Roe, C.A. 133
Rommer, B. 40
Rosen, D.H. 68
Rosing, C. 68–9
Rugg, M.D. 106

Sabom, M. 40, 68, 72, 94, 100
Sachdev, P. 44
Sagan, C. 98
Sanders, A.B. 84
Sartori, P. 90, 130, 131
Schifano, F. 31
Schmidt, D. 82
Schmied, I. 31–2
Schnettler, B. 31–2
Schoenbeck, S. 75

Schontz, F.C. 99
Schwaninger, J. 32, 33, 68
Schwartz, E.K. 132–3
Serdahely, W. 64, 66, 67, 68, 70
Shears, D. 68
Sheeler, R.D. 22
Sherill, E. 17–18
Shushan, G. 117
Singh, C. 55
Sotelo, J. 60
St John of the Cross 119
Stahl, S.M. 114
Stanley, A. 45, 46
Steele, B. 112
Stehle, J.H. 109, 110
Steiger, B. 72
Steiger, S.H. 72
Stevenson, I. 54, 60, 94, 95, 96, 100
Story, F. 58
Strassman, R. 85, 115
Sutherland, C. 14, 60, 65, 68, 70, 71, 72, 73, 74, 75, 76, 78, 125

Tachibana, T. 53
Troscianko, T. 60
Twemlow, S. 45, 64, 66, 71, 94, 99, 125
Tyler, D. 64

Valarino, E.E. 18
van Lommel, P. 15, 18, 19, 32, 33, 34, 36, 42, 44, 46, 48, 56, 68, 89–90, 92, 124, 131
Venecia, D. 64
Verrijp, C.D. 106
Vivien-Roels, B. 110

Walker, B. 64
Wearden, A.J. 133
Whinnery, A.M. 82
Whinnery, J.E. 82
White, R.A. 132
Wickramasinghe, M. 57
Wijethilake, M.M. 60
Wilde, D. 15, 132
Williams Kelly, E. 92
Winkler, E.J. 106, 107
World Health Organization (WHO) 44

Yamamura, H. 52–3
Yanez, J. 109

Zhi-ying, F. 52